COMMUNITY HEALTH AND WELLBEING

Action research on health inequalities

Edited by Steve Cropper, Alison Porter,
Gareth Williams, Sandra Carlisle, Robert Moore,
Martin O'Neill, Chris Roberts and Helen Snooks

First published in Great Britain in 2007 by

The Policy Press
University of Bristol
Fourth Floor
Beacon House
Queen's Road
Bristol BS8 1QU
UK

Tel +44 (0)117 331 4054
Fax +44 (0)117 331 4093
e-mail tpp-info@bristol.ac.uk
www.policypress.org.uk

British Library Cataloguing in Publication Data
A catalogue record for this book is available from the British Library.

Library of Congress Cataloging-in-Publication Data
A catalog record for this book has been requested.

ISBN 978 1 86134 818 0 (paperback)
ISBN 978 1 86134 819 7 (hardback)

Cover design by Qube Design Associates, Bristol.
Front cover: photograph supplied by kind permission of Getty Images
Printed and bound in Great Britain by Cromwell Press, Trowbridge

Contents

Contents

List of tables and figures

Tables

Figures

Preface

The characteristic government approach to reducing the demand on healthcare services is to exhort individuals to change their behaviour, through adopting healthier lifestyles. There are three problems with this approach. First, the growing body of evidence available on health inequalities – evidence that is much more powerful than it was when the Black Report was produced – suggests that what happens 'upstream' is determined by large-scale social and economic forces that are beyond the control of individuals or households. Second, many policies and programmes aimed at changing health behaviour to reduce the risk of later ill health have been successful for some groups in the population but not for others, thus widening the health gap between rich and poor, or between middle class and working class. Third, much poor health is located in particular areas characterised by multiple deprivation and forms of social exclusion. Looked at in this way, many problems that are usually regarded as the responsibility of different departments of government – crime, poor housing, poor educational attainment and chronic ill health – are seen to be interconnected in ways that require the search for 'joined-up' solutions. The search for effective solutions to complex and interconnected problems, or 'wicked issues', has led to a growing emphasis on the need to examine what works: to develop ways of evaluating whether the policies and initiatives in which national and local government invests actually succeed; and to do so in a way that does not add to the sense of exclusion of those who are the targets of the initiatives. This book aims to contribute to that search.

This book is the outcome of an innovative five-year programme to explore the potential of action research as an approach to addressing health inequalities. The Sustainable Health Action Research Programme (SHARP), which was funded by the Welsh Assembly Government through its Health Promotion Division (now the Health Improvement Division), consisted of seven projects. All involved public service agencies, academic institutions and communities as partners, but each was distinctively shaped by its particular sectoral and/or institutional affiliation (health, local government, youth service, further and higher education); the communities it was working with and for (geographical communities, communities of identity, urban/rural); and the forms of investment and intervention chosen by each project.

Activities that came about through SHARP ranged from a travelling information van for young people in rural areas, through the formation of community organisations able to advise on community needs and priorities, to establishment of exercise classes for the over-fifties. In one area, young parents gained formal qualifications in research methods, while in another, community members collected and analysed data for action plans for their communities, to be presented to local policy makers. Some activities had an explicit health focus, such as swimming classes for Asian women and work with children on healthy eating. They were complemented by those that built social networks or social capital through, for example, a film club in a deprived south Wales valleys community, and those that worked to build participants' confidence and self-esteem, such as peer-led dance classes and other activities for young women.

From the point of view of the newly emergent Welsh Assembly, SHARP was a bold experiment; but it is one that very much fitted the ethos, ideology and intent of the Assembly's approach to government in the early years of its existence. All the projects were subject to conventional reporting requirements for the purposes of financial control, policy learning, review and development. But the governance of the projects was undertaken with a remarkably light touch, offering advice and support where necessary, and recognising that all seven projects were complex assemblages whose glitches and hiccoughs could not be governed or managed out of existence. Things did not always run smoothly, nor was it expected that they would.

The Assembly was also very supportive of the widest possible dissemination of findings through academic and professional literatures, and through informal presentations and word-of-mouth conversations within communities. Each project had responsibility for evaluation and for reporting the learning that was attained, but there have also been regular meetings of the seven projects, facilitated by representatives of the Health Promotion Division, and an overarching evaluation project, undertaken by academics at Keele University, to draw out findings from the programme as a whole. Representatives of all of these interests were actively involved in the preparation of this book, for which the Welsh Assembly Government provided support.

Improving health in populations in which health is poor is a complex process. This book argues that the traditional government approach of exhorting individuals to live healthier lifestyles is not enough, and that action to promote public health needs to take place not just through public agencies, but also by engaging community assets and resources in their broadest sense. Complex and sustained community action and effective local partnership are fundamental components of the mix of factors required to address health inequalities successfully. This book reports lessons from the experience of planning, establishing and delivering such action. In particular, the book reports on the potential of an action research approach to developing policy and practice that draws on a range of methods of participatory inquiry. Over a period of five years, the seven projects have investigated both what community health and wellbeing mean in practical terms, and a range of actions to mobilise resources in and for communities affected by inequalities.

The book is organised thematically, with the chapters grouped into three sections. The first section of the book is literature-based. It begins by reviewing the development of understanding of inequalities in health and wellbeing in Britain over the past 25 years. It continues, in the second chapter, by examining the processes by which public policy is created and implemented, and the complex, reciprocal relationship between policy and local circumstances that bring a network of interests into policy making and policy learning. Chapter Three explores the efflorescence in Wales and beyond of a policy environment designed to 'address' health inequalities and related issues, and introduces the seven projects within the Welsh Assembly Government's SHARP programme. In the second section, different dimensions of the SHARP programme are explored in detail, looking at conceptual and methodological questions; issues of organisation and collaboration; and tensions between different stakeholders that emerged through the processes of developing community-based participatory action research. The third section of the book considers learning from the SHARP programme, first in terms of the nature of evidence and the evaluation processes involved, and then by considering what has been learnt about the role of communities in creating and sustaining health. The book's concluding chapter draws key issues together and, in suggesting lessons for national and local policy, provides evidence on how future action on health inequalities might be promoted and strengthened.

Throughout the book, the experience of SHARP and current literature on health inequalities and on action research will be assessed critically in relation to one another. In addition, chapters contain examples and vignettes drawn from the seven SHARP projects to illustrate arguments about theory, method, policy and practice.

While 'health inequality' has established itself in the policy lexicon, its meaning for local policy and practice is still to be elaborated, and policy remains to be developed and refined. In particular, there is still a long way to go in developing strategies for the systematic exploration of which community-based strategies work, and why. The learning from SHARP will be of value to policy makers and practitioners as well as to academics and students interested in health and in public policy. The book does not seek to rehearse analyses of inequality, but, rather, aims to reveal the practicalities of policy implementation – partnership and community involvement – and to assess the value of action research approaches in developing local policy and practice.

An interesting observation about the SHARP programme, which in turn makes the book unusual, is that it takes an approach to research that has conventionally been used in societies without the benefits of the economic and social infrastructure that those working in universities and other professional agencies in the capitalist world take for granted. Moreover, it is an approach that has traditionally been used as the basis of a critique of and a challenge to the existing order, presenting alternative perspectives on reality, giving voice to the voiceless, power to the powerless and so on. In this case, however, the approach has been commissioned by a government department. All sorts of questions arise from this situation: how much control do funders retain over research? What different visions of what can be achieved are held by different players? How are these changed over time? Is it possible to achieve participatory action research in this context and what are the limits to this approach? Who actually sets the agenda in the individual projects? What if the communities had come up with *really* radical suggestions for what they wanted? Do the kind of projects SHARP has been involved in need indefinite public funding? If so, what should the relationship with funders be? Was the Welsh Assembly Government just being cynical and tokenistic in commissioning SHARP? Is the whole programme a modern example of what Herbert Marcuse referred to more than 40 years ago as the 'repressive tolerance' of liberal capitalist societies?

Many of these questions will be addressed in the text, and they are questions that do involve multiple answers; it is for that reason that we have taken a multiple approach to authorship. Authorship in such an enterprise is not straightforward. The editors of this book and the authors of each chapter represent only a part of the human labour that went into the production of the projects on which this book is based. In addition to the co-authors and editorial team, named individually against chapters and/or the book as a whole, we would like to acknowledge the contribution of many others who participated in a variety of ways in SHARP, or in the development of this book.

First and foremost we would like to thank all those who were involved in SHARP projects, at all levels and at all stages. Clearly, without the involvement and cooperation of the people who live and work in areas where the projects took place, there would have been no findings to learn from. We would like to thank the many people who were involved in the research and writing-up process, including Dawn

Armstrong-Esther, Neil Caldwell, Carolyn Lester, Pat Gregory, Deanne Rebane, Jeanne Davies, Roger Beech and Richard Little.

In addition, we gratefully acknowledge the backing of the members of the Welsh Assembly Government, and officers within the Health Promotion Division, in commissioning and supporting the programme and this book to draw together messages and learning from across the programme.

Finally, to all others who have contributed but have not been named – through giving advice, reading sections and helping to move from ideas to initial drafts to the product you now see – we owe a great deal, and offer you our collective thanks. In particular, we thank Michelle Russell, Angela Clements, Nina Parry-Langdon and Kaori Onoda for their contributions in the early stages of drafting and coordinating production of the book across our many co-authors. We would like to thank the numerous people who were key participants in the programme but who have not directly authored the texts of this book; their names are listed in an appendix.

It is easy to dismiss SHARP-style experiments as lacking the hard-nosed rigour of more conventional approaches to evaluation; and as distractions from the real business of improving health through better healthcare delivery and the elimination of unhealthy behaviours wherever they may be found. This default position is very powerful. Unlike hospital waiting times and budgets, health inequalities are not a 'P45' or a 'hanging' issue. Failing to reduce them does not result in mass sackings or executions of managers, doctors or nurses. Nonetheless, what has been easily understood on the streets of Merthyr Tydfil and Pembrokeshire is being gradually and hesitatingly grasped by governments and their civil servants: people make their own history but not under conditions they themselves have chosen. The 'full engagement' in health improvement called for by Derek Wanless as the foundation of sustainable health is a challenge for professionals and agencies at least as much as it is for local communities. The Sustainable Health Action Research Programme in Wales provides important explorations of how this might be possible.

Acknowledgements

Barefoot: Thanks to Jasmin Chowdhury, Tarek Wareth, Musa Yousuf and Edna Esprit-Griffiths and the members of the communities in Butetown, Grangetown and south Cardiff with whom the project worked. Acknowledgement also goes to the project partnership and the public sector and voluntary organisations that they represented.

BeWEHL (Bettws Women's Education, Health and Lifestyle project): In addition to the first co-researchers, Patricia Harris, Andrea Williams, Shelly Wesson, Suzannah Evans and Isabelle Bessant, who provided us with the tools to develop the BeWEHL model, thanks are due to Valerie French, to many of the Bettws community groups and associations, to the partners to the project and to Enid Hankins of the Workers' Educational Association.

Holway: Thanks to Elspeth Morris for her research assistance throughout the project; the many local authority and voluntary sector workers who contributed to the success of the project; and the people of Holway estate.

HYPP (Health of Young People in Powys): Thanks to Brenda Alexander, Dawn Armstrong-Esther, Sue Bayliss, Janet Bidgood, Jenny Bracegirdle, Helen Colby, Anne Davies, Eironwy Davies, Rob Davies, Jenny Deaville, Marnie Garner, Chris Gittoes, Marie Grannell, Angie Heins, Kerry Hodges, Chris Jones, Sioned Jones, Nic Knapton, Carol Morgan, Jenny Lewis and Paul Rowe.

Pembrokeshire: Thanks to the community groups Monkton Voice, CHAD and Llais Llanychaer, which played a key role in the Pembrokeshire SHARP project. Thanks also to the community researchers for their enthusiasm and commitment: Barbara Harries, Shari Jenkins, Angie Meredith, Vanessa Moseley, Tricia Davies, Julie Hicks, Cathy McGrath, Gladys Williams, Roger Griffiths, Miranda Lloyd, Ken Pearson, Sue Russill and Elin Thomas. And thanks to the project's statutory, voluntary and academic partners; to Hayley Thomas and Anna Tee for initiating the project; to Ceri Rothero for design support; and to Diana O'Sullivan for keeping the office in order.

Right 2 Respect, Wrexham: Thanks to Sarah O'Connell, Helen Miller, Nicky Jones, Lowry Kendrick, Beth Parry, Geoff Moore, Andy

Rimmer, Jim Humphries, the young women from the six communities, and youth workers and colleagues in partner agencies involved in the project.

Triangle: Thanks to Neil Caldwell, Jeanne Davies, Pat Gregory, Carolyn Lester and Deanne Rebane for their work on the project; the staff and members of the community associated with the South Riverside Community Development Centre; the 3 Gs Community Centre; Ystradgynlais Volunteer Centre and Ystradgynlais Healthy Living Centre for their participation and involvement; the local health alliances, local health boards and local authorities of Cardiff, Merthyr Tydfil and Powys for their help and support.

Welsh Assembly Government: Thanks to colleagues involved in the development and overall management of SHARP: Launa Anderson, Jan Bunce, Cathryn Gordon, Janine Hale, Ruth Hall, Nina Parry-Langdon, Elaine Mullan, Kaori Onoda and Chris Tudor-Smith.

Overarching evaluation team, Centre for Health Planning and Management, Keele University: Thanks to Dr Roger Beech, Richard Little and Michelle Russell.

Notes on contributors

Bronwen Bermingham has held the post of Project Manager of the 'Barefoot' Health Workers project since 2002. This SHARP-funded project has worked with the Somali, Yemeni and Bangladeshi communities in the Butetown and Grangetown areas of south Cardiff. She is employed by the National Public Health Service and based with the Cardiff Local Public Health Team. With a background in teaching and ESOL (English for speakers of other languages), she has spent most of her working life in the statutory and voluntary sectors. She is interested in the application of organisational and behavioural theory to day-to-day management practice.

Sandra Carlisle has an academic background in medical social anthropology and sociology applied to public health and community health development. She has experience of a wide variety of health-related and policy-relevant research and evaluation projects in both academic and non-academic settings. She is currently Research Fellow in the Public Health Section of the University of Glasgow. Research interests include: sociological and anthropological approaches to understanding health, wellbeing and social inequalities; community health and social inclusion partnerships; community participation in action research; and ethnographic and theory-focused methodologies applied to research and evaluation.

Angela Clements is currently a social researcher at the Office for National Statistics working on design and analysis of social surveys. Previously, she worked as a social researcher in the Public Health Improvement Division (now the Public Health and Health Professions Department) of the Welsh Assembly Government working on research and evaluation to support policy development. This role included working on the SHARP programme, specifically managing the design of action research materials. She has a background in research methods and a particular interest in the way social research can inform and influence the policy-making process, especially with the use of qualitative methodology and analysis.

David Cohen is Professor of Health Economics and Director of the Health Economics and Policy Research Unit at the University of Glamorgan. He has published widely on a variety of issues in health economics. He has been a member of numerous committees and working parties, including the Royal College of Physicians Working Party on Preventative Medicine and the Department of Health Advisory Group on Genetics Research. He has acted as specialist adviser to the World Health Organization and to the House of Commons Select Committee on Welsh Affairs. David has been a member of several research commissioning panels including the MRC Health Service and Public Health Research Board, the NHS Health Technology Assessment R&D Programme, the Wales Office for R&D in Health and Social Care and the National Prevention Research Initiative. In 2002/03 he acted as Deputy Director of the NHS Service Delivery and Organisation R&D Programme and is currently Co-Vice Chair of its Programme Board.

Steve Cropper is Professor of Management in the Centre for Health Planning and Management at Keele University, where he is Director of the Research Institute for Public Policy and Management. He is Chair of the NHS Research for Patient Benefit funding programme for the West Midlands region. He was principal investigator on the overarching evaluation of SHARP. Research interests are inter-organisational collaboration, social capital and community health development; and planning, evaluation and decision support methodologies.

Angela Evans was principal action researcher with the Pembrokeshire SHARP project. She is an experienced community development worker with a particular interest in working with community groups who want to be involved in learning from and evaluating their actions, in order to enhance their participation and ownership. She now works as a researcher for AWARD, the All Wales Alliance for Research and Development in health and social care, based in the School of Medicine at Swansea University. She continues to be interested in participation, public involvement and using collaborative ways of working. She also volunteers within her home community.

Mark Goodwin is Professor of Human Geography at the University of Exeter, and was the academic director of the HYPP SHARP project in Powys. His research has centred on an analysis of the structures and processes of sub-national government, including the recent rise of local and regional partnerships. Empirical work on the changing nature of government has covered the policy areas of housing, health and economic development, and conceptual and theoretical work has helped to elaborate the concepts of local state and local governance. He has written extensively on these subjects in academic journals and has written or edited eight books, including *Introducing Human Geographies* (Arnold, 2005), *Practising Human Geography* (Sage Publications, 2004) and *Envisioning Human Geographies* (Arnold, 2004).

Robert Moore is Emeritus Professor of Sociology at the University of Liverpool. His research career includes writing a number of community studies and publishing work on immigration, race relations and equal opportunities. More recently, he has participated in a number of European-wide projects on labour migration. During the lifetime of SHARP, he produced an atlas of deprivation for Flintshire County Council and he is currently working on census-based research. He was the academic collaborator in the Holway SHARP project in Holywell, North Wales, and lives within walking distance of the estate, where he still acts as an informal adviser to the tenants and residents.

Martin O'Neill had a varied career before entering academia, working as a bus driver, labourer, fence erector and ambulance man among other occupations. He has worked for the Universities of Swansea, Cardiff (where he was the lead researcher on the Triangle project) and Glamorgan. His research interests include health, social and economic regeneration and participatory action research. He is currently Lecturer/Academic Coordinator on the Gates project and Director of the Merthyr Media project. In addition to his role as academic adviser to the North Merthyr Tydfil Regeneration Partnership, he also sits on the management committee of the Merthyr Tydfil Healthy Living Centre.

Janet Pinder is a senior lecturer and research coordinator at the Centre for Community and Lifelong Learning at the University of Wales, Newport. She has managed and coordinated a number of action research-based projects focusing on the impact of learning on health and wellbeing, specifically targeting disadvantaged communities. She was the academic and research lead on the SHARP BeWEHL project. Her research and teaching interests are social inclusion and social equity, community development, and efficacy.

Alison Porter is a researcher for AWARD. She is based in the School of Medicine at Swansea University, which was one of the partners in the Pembrokeshire SHARP project. She is interested in processes of participation and other aspects of the relationship between organisations and people who use their services. As well her research interests, she has practical experience of working in the voluntary and statutory sectors on community development and service planning. Alison Porter was funded by the Welsh Assembly Government to coordinate production of this book.

Chris Roberts is a social researcher in the Public Health and Health Professions Department, Welsh Assembly Government. He is responsible for commissioning research and evaluation to support policy development and leads the team that developed and managed the SHARP project in Wales. He has a particular interest in the evaluation of interventions designed to improve public health, encouraging a range of methodologies and disciplinary approaches.

Kevin Shales is a community development officer with Pembrokeshire County Council. He was an action researcher working on the Pembrokeshire SHARP project. He then went on to undertake a community consultation process, following the principles of the Pembrokeshire SHARP model, for Pembrokeshire County Council's Social Care and Housing Directorate. This explored how older residents could remain living more independently in their own homes. His particular interest is the welfare and best interests of disabled children and their families. He has worked as a research therapist, studying treatments for cerebral palsy in China and Australia.

Helen Snooks is Professor of Health Services Research, based in the Centre for Health Information, Research and Evaluation in the School of Medicine at Swansea University. She is currently Director of AWARD's Mid and West Wales section. Her main research interests and expertise lie in the fields of emergency and unscheduled care, participatory research and research support. In these areas, she plans, designs and carries out service user-focused evaluations of new models of service delivery, which often involve changing roles and working across boundaries between service providers.

Gareth Williams is Professor of Sociology in the School of Social Sciences at Cardiff University. He is Director of the Welsh Health Impact Assessment Support Unit, Associate Director of the Cardiff Institute of Society, Health and Ethics, Deputy Director of the Regeneration Institute, and Chair of AWARD. He was principal investigator on the Triangle project within the SHARP programme. His particular interests are in inequality, social deprivation, regeneration, long-term illness and incapacity, and the sociology of knowledge and expertise.

ONE

Health inequalities in their place

Gareth Williams

Introduction

A great deal has changed since the publication of Sir Douglas Black's ground-breaking report on inequalities in health (DHSS, 1980). In response to an article published in the now defunct *New Society* magazine (Wilkinson, 1976), the report was commissioned by the Secretary of State for Health and Social Services in 1977, during the dying days of James Callaghan's Labour government, in an economic environment characterised by deep cuts in public expenditure, sharply rising unemployment and growing industrial unrest. The Black Report finally entered the public domain in the bright light of a new Conservative dawn in British politics. 'Published' over a Bank Holiday weekend in 1980 in the form of 260 photocopies, the report would have disappeared from view had it not been for the tenacity of the report's authors, and the support of activists within the public health movement. Later published as a Penguin paperback (Townsend et al, 1988), alongside an important update from the Health Education Council (Whitehead, 1987), the Black Report was initially disseminated by being passed among friends and sympathisers, in the manner of Mikhail Bulgakov's *The Master and Margarita* and other post-Stalin, Soviet-bloc *samizdat* literature.

The class conflict, ideological divisions and social polarisation that characterised British society throughout the 1980s made it difficult to conduct any reasoned discussion of the nature of the evidence and arguments contained in the Black Report (Macintyre, 1997). The Black Report itself had been very firm in its view that health inequalities existed, and that structural or material factors provided the best explanation of them. Subsequent arguments became entrenched in debates over whether or not health inequalities really did exist and, if they did, whether it was because less healthy people were more likely to become poor, or because of patterns of individual behaviour in different socioeconomic groups, or something – social structure, or material conditions – over which individual people had little if no control (Bloor et al, 1987;Vågerö and Illsley, 1995).The cross-sectional nature of much of the data on which the Black Report was based made it difficult to resolve some of these disagreements.What was also clear, however, was that Margaret Thatcher and her ministers were not in a receptive frame of mind and, with an intuitive understanding of the power of language, Conservative governments spent the next 15 years assiduously avoiding the use of the term 'inequality', apparently hoping that this would make inequalities disappear, at least as far as public debate was concerned. In short, the ideological climate was increasingly inhospitable to the Black Report's basic assumptions and precepts.

The contrast with the later Acheson Report (Acheson, 1998) could not be greater. Commissioned by and published under the official auspices of a 'New Labour' government on the rise, the findings of the report provided an update of the Black Report.While reinforcing the fundamentals of Black's materialistic message, the report also had the benefit of a range of new and more sophisticated data sets than those available to Black, and a less fraught ideological environment. It was therefore able to tailor and refine its explanations for what was to be done. Perhaps because of the rather more relaxed ideological environment, the Acheson Report produced a new and important summary of the state of knowledge of health inequalities, but it was relatively unfocused, both in its theoretical analysis and in its policy recommendations, with no attempt to prioritise these or to place a monetary value against them.

In this chapter, we review some of the contemporary evidence and discuss the way in which new evidence has allowed for the development of much more subtle and fine-grained approaches to the process of explaining health inequalities. We discuss the relationship between health status and health services, and the way in which a partial rehabilitation of the concept of society since Margaret Thatcher has created space for a more creative relationship between the social sciences and the politics of health inequalities. This sets the scene for the discussion of policy innovation in Chapters Two and Three.

Health inequalities

The overall sociodemographic picture in Britain and elsewhere throughout the 20th century, as McKeown (1979) brilliantly if controversially argued, is of improving economic and social conditions leading to increasing life expectancy and population growth, with public health interventions and medical care playing a distinctly supporting role. In the wake of improvements in infant and child health, death rates have been halved and life expectancy has risen. This improvement has continued throughout the 21st century. Between 1971 and 2003, life expectancy for men increased from 69.1 to 76.2 years and for women from 75.3 to 80.5 years (ONS, 2005). In the 21st century, it is chronic, degenerative conditions such as heart disease, cancer and stroke that dominate the mortality statistics; and these, along with diabetes, musculoskeletal disorders, chronic respiratory diseases and mental health problems, are also responsible for high rates of long-term illness and disability in some population groups. In spite of overall improvements in health, the unequal distribution of ill health is a continuing and growing feature (Shaw et al, 2007). By 2003, there was a gap in estimated life expectancy between professional and unskilled manual social classes of over eight years for men and almost five years for women (ONS, 2005). Moreover, in terms of the social ecology of health of whole societies, in developed societies levels of health seem to be driven less by overall levels of income and wealth and more by economic inequalities within the society (Wilkinson, 1996; 2005).

One of the crucial arguments to be developed since the Black Report is that while inequalities in health can be seen in terms of the disadvantages of simply being poor, they can also be seen in relation to the 'health gap' between rich and poor, or the 'health gradient' that tracks socioeconomic position across the population (Graham, 2004). The concept of the gradient means that there is an increased risk of premature mortality on each step down the class ladder, and this is the case for women as for men (Graham, 2001). If you take coronary heart disease, the single major cause of death in the UK, death rates among men are approximately 40 per cent higher for manual workers than for non-manual workers; and the death rate for female partners of manual workers is about twice the rate for those of non-manual workers (Marmot, 1998). In economically developed societies, the importance of the class gradient, and relative differences between groups, as opposed to absolute poverty or wealth, has been illustrated very powerfully by the work of Marmot and his colleagues on British civil servants working in Whitehall, who were followed up 25 years after data collection first began (Marmot and Shipley, 1996).

Within the UK, inequalities in health by social position, whether measured in terms of income and wealth or occupation, or indeed length of education or the quality of housing, are reiterated in regional mortality and morbidity (Boyle et al, 2004). Maps of regional mortality in the UK show that the spatial patterning of health is repeated at area level (Graham, 2001), with high premature mortality in the post-industrial regions of central Scotland (most notoriously, 'the

Glasgow effect'), Northern Ireland, north-west and north-east England, inner London and the valleys of south Wales (Shaw et al, 1999). In view of the focus of the Welsh Assembly Government's Sustainable Health Action Research Programme (SHARP), it is pertinent to say something specifically about Wales itself, an identity that is often lost in the tendency to look at statistics for 'England and Wales', or indeed to pretend that Wales does not exist. In Wales, as elsewhere, mortality has fallen steadily since the 1980s, including mortality from major causes of death such as cancers and circulatory diseases; and men have higher death rates and shorter life expectancy than women (Higgs et al, 1998). Infant mortality rates fell until the early 1990s but have fluctuated since (Chief Medical Officer, 2003), with figures for 1999 showing a higher rate in Wales than in Scotland or England. In broad terms, taking age-standardised mortality rates as the measure of overall health in the population, the health of the people of Wales is worse than that in England, but slightly better than Scotland and broadly similar to Northern Ireland. Life expectancy is two or three years shorter than the best in Europe and death rates are relatively high. Figures for 1998 show life expectancy in Wales to be 74.5 years for men and 79.5 years for women, the same as for Northern Ireland (Gordon et al, 2001).

The most striking data emerge from comparisons between localities within the country. By 2003, the gap between the best and the worst local authority areas was almost 12 years (ONS, 2005). These differences are most often defined in relation to local authority boundaries, but it is important to bear in mind that there are often 'hidden' differences within such areas that are as great as the visible differences between them. Mortality rates for particular post-industrial communities may be higher than other 'similar' communities a relatively short distance away. In general, however, overall, age-standardised mortality rates are higher in the south Wales valley areas of Merthyr Tydfil, Blaenau Gwent, Caerphilly and Rhondda Cynon Taff, and lower in the more rural areas of Ceredigion, Monmouthshire and Powys. Merthyr Tydfil, the unitary authority area with the highest rates, has mortality rates 50 per cent higher than the area with the lowest rates, Ceredigion. Life expectancy is 71.1 years in Merthyr Tydfil and 76.1 years in Ceredigion. While the mortality figures in the worst parts of Wales are not quite as bad as those of the worst Scottish areas, nonetheless the life expectancy figures in the worst local authority areas in Wales in the period 1995–97 had not reached the UK average for 1986 (Gordon et al, 2001). If you look at potential years of life lost, rural areas with high injury rates (often related to agricultural work) such as Denbighshire have high rates of potential years lost, but Merthyr Tydfil remains the worst on this measure too, with rates in Monmouthshire being about 50 per cent lower. This kind of poor health in particular localities is not new, with Merthyr Tydfil and Rhondda, for example, often being cited in historical accounts (Williams, 1998; Smith, 1999).

Wales has very high rates of limiting long-term illness (LLTI) compared with the rest of the UK, higher even than Scotland, in spite of the higher mortality rates in Scotland, and this is true across all age groups. Prevalence of LLTI is particularly high in coalfield areas everywhere, higher than inner London areas and rivalled only by old port and industrial areas (Joshi et al, 2001). However, the rates of long-term and limiting long-term illness in Wales are higher than you would predict on the basis of mortality rates. The LLTI rates are particularly high in the post-industrial world of the south Wales valleys. At county/regional level, Mid Glamorgan, West Glamorgan and Gwent have the highest rates of LLTI in Britain. At the level of district authorities, based on 1991 data, seven of the 10 highest scoring districts are in south Wales. When the 1991 data are analysed at the level of wards and 'pseudo postcode sectors', 15 of the top 20 areas are in Wales (14 in south Wales, one in Wrexham in north-east Wales), with communities such as Maerdy (Rhondda), Bettws (Ogwr), Pen-y-Waun (Cynon Valley) and Gurnos (Merthyr Tydfil) scoring particularly highly. Analysis of the 2001 Census indicates broadly the same league table, with the only challenge to this undesirable Welsh dominance coming from Easington in county Durham, a former coalmining area in north-east England. The lowest rates are in Guildford, Chichester and other towns in southern England.

Six of the 10 worst areas for LLTI in 2001 are in south Wales, with Merthyr Tydfil, along with Easington, recording 30 per cent or more of the population having some kind of LLTI. Reports of LLTI are more likely among people with heart disease, respiratory illness, mental illness, back pain or arthritis. While rates of LLTI are high across Wales compared with elsewhere in the UK, within Wales there is a difference of more than 10 percentage points between the worst and the best local authority areas (National Assembly for Wales, 2003). These very high rates of LLTI in Wales are repeated for other measures with 15 per cent or more of the populations of Merthyr Tydfil, Blaenau Gwent, Neath-Port Talbot, Rhondda Cynon Taf and Caerphilly reporting their general health as 'not good', and the same areas getting higher scores (worse health) on the SF-36 health status questions. In the Communities First area of Gurnos in Merthyr Tydfil (one of the sites for the SHARP Triangle project), 59.1% of households have one or more persons with an LLTI, compared with 42.4% in Wales as a whole;

and 21.6% of the population describe themselves as 'not being in good health' compared with 12.5% in Wales (Welsh Assembly Government, 2006). The same six Welsh local authority districts mentioned above rank in the top 10 for self-reports of general health not being good and for the percentages of those of working age who are unable to work and claiming benefit for permanent sickness or disability (National Assembly for Wales, 1999).

Social determinants: explaining health inequalities

Although inequalities in the rates of disease and death have been observed in the population of the UK since the great reform movements of the 19th century, the modern debate on health inequalities dates from the publication of the Black Report, discussed earlier. That report showed in one volume for the first time the huge disparities in the chances of long life and good health for different groups in the population of the UK.

Data displaying the social class gradient in such a comprehensive form were powerful enough, though the cross-sectional nature of the data on which it was based opened Black's report to criticism as it attempted to explain the differences observed and suggest policies for action. What was important about the Black Report was that it took the debate beyond singular explanations for differential health risks, such as smoking or employment, and tried to build different categories of explanation, focusing on how the consistent class gradient could be explained. Black and his colleagues identified four possible types of explanation of social inequalities in health: measurement artefact; natural or social selection; materialist-structuralist; and cultural-behavioural. Black's committee, and other commentators, came down firmly in favour of explanations of the materialist or structuralist type. Only these explanations, it was argued, could simultaneously account for the improvements in the general health of the population and the maintenance of class differences in health. The primacy of some kind of materialist framework was later reviewed and supported by Whitehead (1987). While the possibility that the size of the class gradient was an artefact of the measurement process itself was a real one at the time Black reported, more recent evidence indicates that socioeconomic differences in health and the class gradient are very real indeed (Davey Smith et al, 1994). The social selection explanations – that social position is in some way determined by health, rather than vice versa – have been similarly refuted, except as components in an overall analysis of life-course effects (Power et al, 1996).

While there is clear evidence that smoking is a risk factor for early death, neither smoking nor other individual risks such as high cholesterol or blood pressure adequately explain differences in mortality (Shaw et al, 1999). Lifestyles have continued to be the focus for national strategies of health improvement, but they explain a relatively small proportion of the health inequalities between different socioeconomic groups (Graham, 2001). Notwithstanding the prima facie plausibility of cultural and behavioural factors, the key to explaining differences in both behaviour and health outcomes does seem to lie in what are referred to as structural or material factors, primarily those associated with poverty and deprivation arising from socioeconomic position and broader social conditions. These factors may be understood both as hazards inherent in society that have a direct impact on health, and as the conditions that create unhealthy behaviours, and make behaviour change in response to public health advice less likely. Material and what are sometimes called 'neo-material' factors (Bartley, 2004) include the physical environment in the home, neighbourhood and workplace, and the living standards secured through earnings, benefits and other sources of income.

In recent times, the availability of richer data sources and innovative techniques of analysis, as well as the development of new theoretical perspectives on the relationships between individual lives and social structures, have opened different ways of thinking about these questions (Bartley, 2004). Although Dahlgren and Whitehead's (Dahlgren and Whitehead, 1991), well-known 'rainbow' diagram of the determinants of health is largely a descriptive aide-memoire, it suggests that a primary emphasis on wider, possibly global, socioeconomic determinants does not exclude consideration of the effects of regional and local social infrastructure, neighbourhood, households and individuals. In contrast to the debate between the materialists and the individualists post-Black, the key message is that while individual behaviour may have some explanatory importance, it cannot be understood in any meaningful way outside the other layers of the rainbow. These ideas have been applied both to the unequal distribution of health between different socioeconomic groups, and to the determinants of health in whole populations (Wilkinson, 1996; Bartley, 2004; Wilkinson, 2005).

Moreover, difficulties and problems can build up over time, exposing people to different kinds of risks and benefits at different points in the cycle or course of life – the way in which '... advantages and disadvantages tend to cluster cross-sectionally and accumulate longitudinally' (Blane, 1999, p 64). This kind of perspective has led to an increasing emphasis on looking at inequalities in health in different areas, where the combined effects of the composition of populations and the context of areas can be examined. At an individual level, the cross-generational and cumulative effects of poverty and disadvantage have been shown in the effects of maternal malnourishment and low birth-weight over time (Davey Smith and Kuh, 1997). These processes clearly involve complex interaction between socioeconomic, biological and behavioural factors over the life course. The cumulative effects of area histories have been less well explored, but given the increasing evidence of dramatic area variations in mortality and morbidity that appear to be in part related to area characteristics (context), in addition to the characteristics of the individuals living in those areas (composition), the cumulative effects of economic disinvestments and social decline over generations are important parts of a fuller sociological picture (Joshi et al, 2001), not least in some Welsh regions with a rise, fall and partial regeneration that has been so dramatically compressed in time (Smith, 1993).

These new developments in thinking have led to arguments for more detailed research into the 'black box' of materialist explanations for health inequalities. The continued existence and indeed widening of the health gap between wealthier and poorer people, and between advantaged and disadvantaged areas, raises all kinds of questions about the relationship between people and the social conditions in which they live and work. In order to move beyond simple restatements of the Black Report's judgements on poverty, or common-sense descriptions of unhealthy behaviours, more imaginative approaches to theory and evidence are needed.

Inside the black box: interpreting health inequalities

It is increasingly argued that conventional approaches to the explanation of social inequalities in health have created a 'black box', the inputs and outputs to and from which we can observe, measure and correlate, but whose interior workings – how inequality, poverty, and powerlessness affect health in different social contexts – remain obscure, partly because of their resistance to easy epidemiological examination (Shim, 2002). Understanding health inequalities additionally requires a 'more micro-level examination of the pathways by which social structure actually influences mental and physical health and functioning and life expectancy', and this means adopting a 'more fine-grained' approach (Macintyre, 1997, pp 736-7). This approach will need not just more and better statistical data and tools, but more interpretative and historical approaches, bringing together the stories of individuals and the histories of social structures in particular areas – cities, towns and communities (Popay et al, 1998). Communities, like individuals, accumulate advantages and disadvantages over time. Inside the occasionally convoluted theorising of the late Pierre Bourdieu is a simple message – 'the social world is accumulated history' (1986, p 241) – and the stories about the 'weight of the world' (Bourdieu et al, 1999) hammer home the point that structure can be very heavy indeed, undermining individual and collective capacities and capabilities. Rather than thinking of health simply in terms of class or socioeconomic position, the focus on communities and neighbourhoods encourages a multidimensional approach to the forms of 'social suffering' characteristic of later modernity. As Blackman has argued:

> Places matter because they are open, dynamic and adaptive systems that do not have a simple cause-effect relationship with national or global drivers of economic, social or policy change. (Blackman, 2006, p 1)

Although poverty, inequality and other economic indicators of social development may remain the 'base' condition underlying health inequalities, the 'superstructure' is not irrelevant. The political and cultural responses to economic conditions have themselves 'multiplied the social spaces ... and set up the conditions for an unprecedented development of all kinds of ordinary suffering' (Bourdieu, 1999, p 4).

In trying to think of practical ways in which such an approach could be developed, we need to distinguish between 'material' (de-contextualised) and 'materialist' (contextualised) explanations (Macintyre, 1997). Drawing on this distinction, it has recently been argued that:

> What is missing is a discussion of the relationship between agency (the ability for people to deploy a range of causal powers), practices (the activities that make and transform the world we live in) and social structure (the rules and resources in society). Without such an understanding, factors associated with people's disease experiences within a context tend to be denuded of social meaning. (Frohlich et al, 2001)

There have been a number of studies that have attempted to understand the dynamics of neighbourhoods in terms of networks, social capital and social cohesion, and in doing so to try to understand the social context within which human agency and practices are shaped and in turn allows people to have some impact on social structures (Cattell, 2001; Popay et al, 2003a).These studies have shown how the epidemiological separation of 'context' and 'composition' undermines our ability to understand how people make places and places make people. It constrains our attempts to see places as 'dynamic systems', in Blackman's (2006) terms, not least because they strip the place and the people of any historical referent. Those places that are now regarded as vales of tears were, no more than a hundred years ago, busy 'building Jerusalem' (Pope, 1998). These historical dynamics of place are important determinants of contemporary health inequalities (Williams, 2003).

How might a more dynamic analysis make sense in the context of the poor health of people in socially deprived communities in Wales? And how might this analysis inform policy and action? There are, of course, many different kinds of regions and localities in Wales. The south Wales former coalfield region can be used here to illustrate the theoretical arguments. In 1998, a report from the Coalfields Task Force argued that coalfield areas had a 'unique combination of concentrated joblessness, physical isolation, poor infrastructure and severe health problems' (Coalfields Task Force, 1998, para 1.2).While it is important to keep the harsh generic reality of material deprivation in the forefront of any explanation of health inequalities in Wales, it is also important to recognise the way in which the particular context of Welsh economic and social history has shaped the people who live in certain parts of it. The bullet-point description provided by the Coalfields Task Force disguises a more complex narrative:

> [In South Wales] this was not just a case of localised economic decline but rather one of cultural crisis. The collapse of coalmining undermined a range of mechanisms of social regulation that were grounded in the politics of the workplace and trades unions, but spread more widely into local society and politics. There was an acute sense of loss in places in which coal mines closed after decades of existence. This was typically accompanied by a period of grieving as people in these places tried to come to terms with the manifold implications of the precipitate ending of the economic raison d'être of their place. (Bennett et al, 2000, p 5)

While the coalmining industry in Wales had been in a state of continuous decline in the period after the Second World War, the combined economic, political and social consequences of the end of the strike of 1984-85 have had an impact on south Wales, the shock of which continues to reverberate through economy, society and culture 20 years on (Williams, 2006).

There are other contemporary examples of the way in which observable and measurable events, such as joblessness and poor housing, become episodes in the histories of places and people. Blaenau Gwent contains areas of severe deprivation, all of whose electoral wards are ranked within the 40 per cent most deprived wards in Wales – Nantyglo, Tredegar Central and West, Llanhilleth, Sirhowy and many others. It has among the lowest levels of earnings and house prices in Britain, a large percentage of the population with no qualifications and, as has been indicated, high levels of long-term ill health. Moreover, with low car ownership and limited access to public transport, the prospects of commuting to work are limited. Following a major strategic review in February 2001, Corus plc announced that it was going to restructure its steel enterprise and industry in Wales. One of the major casualties of this restructuring was the Ebbw Vale steelworks, situated at the heart of the Blaenau Gwent economy, which has now closed.

Developing our understanding of the connections between large-scale social and economic processes requires an imaginative grasp of how things are seen from the points of view of those who have been affected. In research undertaken as part of an examination of the impact of the steel closures in Ebbw Vale (Fairbrother and Morgan, 2001), interviews were carried out with a number of people living and working in the area about what was happening to the people in the locality. These people were not themselves steelworkers, but residents of a locality in which steel had been central. One health visitor working in the area said:

> "People talk not only about the effect on individuals; it's the effect on the borough – everybody, regardless of whether they are employed by Corus or not. I think that there is a huge concern ... that in an area that appeared to be going downhill anyway this is the final nail in the coffin."

The nature of the work and its dominant relationship to the community – in coal and steel – generated powerful social solidarity. As the major industries have withdrawn from Blaenau Gwent, the social and physical landscape has changed: "Abertillery breaks my heart," said the same health visitor, "because it just was not like it looks now, it's just a dump." Many respondents talked about the way in which the running down of the steel works, as well as the mines, affected the way in which local people interacted with each other. Solidarity extended beyond the work into the 'social capital' of the local community. An educational welfare officer recounted:

> "The changes in the area over the past 30 years have been tremendous. It has a feeling all of its own 30 years ago, a very strong community of miners and steelworkers ... and now that's gone."

A district nurse who had always worked in the area spoke in similar terms, drawing attention to the impact of these changes on structures of feeling:

> "That sort of comradeship has all gone. You knew who you could trust and everyone would help you, but that is disappearing, that sort of feeling is disappearing."

The nature of the work defined the kind of relationships that emerged: the communities, the politics and the aesthetics. The sights, sounds and smells associated with the steelworks imprinted themselves on the social and physical character of the surrounding towns. We see in these excerpts from interviews an understanding of the interweaving of personal narratives and social history. Whereas in the past solidarity provided the basis for union and political action, the decline over 30 years and more has created a situation in which the resources for hope and resistance are depleted.

During the course of the interviews, one church minister said:

> "In the space of six months about two years ago I buried five drug-related [deaths]. The youngest was 18 [years of age] and the oldest was a 27-year-old mother who lived in one of the streets up here. And I knew her parents fairly well, and she left a three-year old boy for her parents to look after. It's a very, very, very real problem."

Poverty, inequality, social exclusion – however the distribution of resources and opportunities is conceptualised – have direct consequences for individual lives: educational failure, crime, heart disease, drugs and alcohol. Things – relationships, roles, jobs, thoughts, actions – are fractured and fragmented, no longer making sense in terms of what people understand from past experience. What the church minister spoke about was a sense of people hurtling away from each other in a process of fragmentation, personal expressions of the social conditions underlying many of the problems people face. These narrative fragments were framed within an historical analysis of decline, providing a rich context for our understanding of the way in which ill health is determined by social forces and people's responses to it.

While contemporary indicators of material disadvantage are clearly crucial, the routes through which these affect behaviour and health can be seen in the extent to which people can construct a sense of identity and purpose under very difficult social and economic conditions (Popay et al, 2003a). While the epidemiological distinction between context and composition is a useful way of enhancing our understanding of the clustering of disadvantages, it can also obscure the complex conjoint influence of people and places in determining health outcomes (Smith and Easterlow, 2005). This kind of intertwining of people and place can be seen in the quotations from the people of Blaenau Gwent above.

It is not a question of converting this exploratory historical sociology into epidemiology – we already have good social epidemiology – but rather of developing these impressions into fuller sociological and historical analyses of the interrelationships between people and places over time, and using this to frame or contextualise, inter alia, patterns of health behaviour, health outcomes and appropriate professional and political responses to them (Williams, 2003). What the material referred to in this section shows is that the relationships between structures, contexts and everyday lives are interwoven in complex ways. While behavioural interventions delivered through health services may be part of the policy solution to the problems of poor health in these areas, there is clearly something profoundly limited about treating the lives of individuals in this way, and it is unlikely to be successful in the longer term. What we actually need in thinking about public health is a much more radical point of departure that starts with the 'agent in its environment' engaged in a process of becoming, as opposed to some variation on the idea of a 'petrified' self-contained individual confronting a world 'outside' (Ingold, 2000).

Developing meaningful policy responses

The conventional approach to thinking about health improvement is to argue the case for more and better health services, pointing out that there is, famously, an 'inverse care law': the availability and accessibility of services varies inversely with the need for it in the population served (Hart, 1971). However, while few would want to argue the case against a more equitable distribution of and access to services, the incontestable conclusion to any rigorous review and interpretation of the evidence on health inequalities is that 'most of the major drivers of population health and of the distribution of health lie outside the NHS' (Macintyre,

2000, p 1399). When the world price of steel falls in the context of a strong domestic currency, thousands of people across Wales lose their jobs in places that have already experienced years of relentless de-industrialisation – not something that doctors, nurses, social workers or health and social care managers can do very much about. But these economic and social changes do have consequences for physical and mental health that those health professionals and managers are expected to be able to do something about. The dilemma for those concerned with the people's health and wellbeing is that the more it is shown that variation in morbidity and mortality is associated with social factors of the kind described here, the more it seems that health services of themselves can have little relevance (Blaxter, 1996).

The post-Thatcherite Labour governments and their official advisers in the UK have tended to respond to this dilemma in two ways: first, by acknowledging (in a way Conservative governments were unwilling to do) the importance of large-scale economic, social and environmental determinants of health and health inequalities; and second, by emphasising (as Conservative governments were keen to do) an approach that seeks to persuade, exhort or cajole individuals (or communities understood as aggregations of individuals) to follow 'healthy lifestyles', supported by the 'delivery' of 'interventions' for smoking cessation, alcohol reduction, dietary change and sexual restraint. Although there remains a communitarian gloss on some of the policy documents emerging from New Labour in the UK (DH, 1999), in practical terms the focus has remained firmly on people 'at risk' because of the lifestyles they 'adopt' (Macintyre, 2000). There has been less evidence of sustained *sociological* thinking about the distribution of health risks in terms of how to improve the opportunity structures in local communities and environments – good housing, safe play areas, accessible and reasonably priced food, education and employment opportunities. This paradox makes current approaches to both healthcare delivery and health promotion unsustainable, inequitable and potentially de-stabilising and de-legitimating for welfare states. Sustained thinking of this kind is important both as a corrective to a simplistic emphasis on individual behaviour as *the* problem, and as a contribution to developing a health service agenda that helps to support Wanless' 'fully engaged scenario' (Wanless, 2004).

Within its currently limited powers, the Welsh Assembly Government has been innovative both in its attempts to define new parameters for the development of health policy and in its support for new health developments and initiatives. Since 1998, the Welsh Office and then the Assembly have been involved in a process of responding to the evidence on what determines good and bad health by developing a vision and strategy for improvements in health and wellbeing (Welsh Office, 1998). To its credit, the Assembly has strenuously insisted on placing health within a broader policy context, emphasising the need to '... build bridges between organizations and sectors for more joint action to increase well-being across communities' (Welsh Assembly Government, 2002, p 5).

In the context of an identification of both inequalities in health experience and inequities in the distribution, access and quality of services (National Assembly for Wales, 2001a), the Welsh Assembly Government has promulgated a radical plan for health services in Wales:

> The Assembly has developed ... a number of strategies to counteract social exclusion and to create a *socially inclusive* Wales. It recognises the importance of building and supporting strong *communities* where the values of *citizenship* and collective action can grow....This (Health) Plan builds on wide consultation over the elements that make it up and is part of the process of replacing elite policy making by *participative* policy development. Our policy here is to build on this commitment and to continue to *enhance the citizen's voice* at the heart of policy. (National Assembly for Wales, 2001b, p 5, emphasis in original)

In spite of increasing pressure to do something about waiting times for hospital treatment (that is, to be more like England), an issue that led to the 'reshuffling' of a long-standing health and social services minister, the Assembly has continued to insist on the need to develop a sustainable health policy that refocuses on primary care, prevention and health promotion, and to put in place a formula for the equitable distribution of NHS resources to the new local health boards. This approach has been supported by an external review, conducted by a project team advised by Derek Wanless, which has further emphasised the need for 'a strategic adjustment of services to focus them on prevention and early intervention [entailing] adjusted roles for primary, secondary and social care' (Welsh Assembly Government, 2003b, p 51). While recognising the continuing need for good secondary and tertiary services to deal effectively with ill health, and for urgent action on waiting lists in the short term, Wanless argues that this can only be done sustainably by looking at new models of care as whole systems that can integrate resources across different health and social care sectors.

Like other government advisers before him, Wanless also emphasises that health is too big a problem for the health and social care services alone, and that a 'step-change in individuals' and communities' acceptance of responsibility for their health is needed' (Welsh Assembly Government, 2003b, p 51). However, although in his Welsh review, and elsewhere (Wanless, 2004), Wanless recognises the importance of 'the range of factors which affect health', there is a tendency for the overwhelming determinants of health of the kind described in this chapter to become reduced to rather residual notions of 'personal circumstances' and 'social norms'. We have to move 'beyond beer, fags, egg and chips' (Popay et al, 2003b). The way forward involves the redistribution of opportunities and resources through macro-level policies but, more than this, we need a social movement with a political programme that is genuinely participative, building on the abundant social and cultural resources of 'lay knowledge' (Popay et al, 1998) or 'civic intelligence' (Elliott and Williams, 2003) that exist in local communities and organisations, as well as the considerable social scientific knowledge about the complex effects of social inequalities in health over time and space.

Conclusion

In Wales, as elsewhere, community regeneration or 'neighbourhood renewal' and tackling health inequalities involve interventions in 'wicked' issues or problems (Hunter, 2003). These issues are wicked because they push against the dividing walls of different academic disciplines and because they cut across the boundaries of government departments and budgets, and they are therefore issues for which any one government minister is reluctant to accept responsibility. They are all the more wicked when they are understood to be profoundly interrelated. Strategies for tackling health inequalities cannot work without some kind of intervention in neighbourhoods to tackle the local expressions and manifestations of the structural inequalities that produce poor health and inequalities in health (Blackman, 2006). The effect of neighbourhoods on health includes traditional physical features of neighbourhoods, such as the quality of local housing, the forms of housing tenure and their relationship to local economic resources; the connections between where people live and the availability and accessibility of opportunities, services and facilities; and what is sometimes referred to in rather arcane terms as 'ontological security', or feeling of 'home'.

A formal evaluation of a complex intervention creates all kind of difficulties (Barnes et al, 2005). Some of these difficulties are of a methodological kind, but in interventions where partnership, public involvement and local activity are part of the constitution of the evaluation itself, it does not make any sense to reduce measurement of its worth to traditional methodological criteria. Taking the Health Action Zone evaluation in England as an example, the 'kaleidoscope of local activity' was a strength of the initiative (Judge and Bauld, 2005, p 189), but local direction of priorities and activities makes evaluation as it is normally understood very difficult (Blackman, 2006). As Robert Moore describes it in Chapter Eight of this volume, although the closeness of intervention and evaluation makes traditional evidence-based statements of effect difficult, the action research methodology allowed the researchers to observe close up the complex and dynamic interrelationships of the acquisition of new skills, the growth of self-esteem and self-confidence, and the way in which this built different kinds of capital within the communities.

In Wales, SHARP worked with broad definitions of both intervention and outcome, and can be seen, perhaps, as a 'systematic exploration' rather than a formal evaluation of what works. As we argue later, the SHARP projects can perhaps be more adequately conceptualised as exercises in 'demonstrable rationality' (Marris and Rein, 1974), combining evidence, general academic expertise, professional judgement and forms of lay knowledge in complex ways that do not fit easily within conventional notions of 'evidence-based'. In combining the external expertise of non-local agencies such as universities with the internal expertise of local community members and agencies, the projects in SHARP were able to look at *what works* in the context of *what matters*. By bringing academic health experts together with local agencies and communities, within an action research framework, SHARP set out to explore new ways in which community-based programmes, involving local people and local professional agencies, can make some contribution to improving health in a sustainable way.

In the next two chapters, we explore ways in which the policy challenge of health inequalities has been conceptualised and implemented, looking at forms of policy initiative and action. The first chapter, by Steve Cropper and Mark Goodwin, examines the nature of public policy and the ways in which it is made in response to the issues of need and welfare that we currently face. The chapter that follows focuses on the Welsh context in which SHARP was developed, and connects it to the wider issues discussed by Cropper. These three chapters together provide the conceptual foundation for exploring the ways in which key issues relating to community-based interventions were handled and developed in the context of the SHARP projects.

References

Acheson, D. (1998) *Independent Inquiry into Inequalities in Health: Report*, London: HMSO.

Barnes, M., Bauld, L., Benzeval, M., Judge, K., Mackenzie, M. and Sullivan, H. (2005) *Health Action Zones: Partnerships for Health Equity*, London: Routledge.

Bartley, M. (2004) *Health Inequalities: An Introduction to Theories, Concepts and Methods*, Cambridge: Polity Press.

Bennett, K., Beynon, H. and Hudson, R. (2000) *Coalfields Regeneration: Dealing with the Consequences of Industrial Decline*, Bristol: Policy Press.

Blackman, T. (2006) *Placing Health: Neighbourhood Renewal, Health Improvement and Complexity*, Bristol: Policy Press.

Blane, D. (1999) 'The life course, the social gradient and health', in M. Marmot and R.G. Wilkinson (eds) *Social Determinants of Health*, Oxford: Oxford University Press.

Blaxter, M. (1996) 'The significance of socioeconomic factors in health for medical care and the National Health Service', in D. Blane, E. Bruner and R. Wilkinson (eds) *Health and Social Organization*, London: Routledge, pp 32-41.

Bloor, M., Samphier, M. and Prior, L. (1987) 'Artefact explanations of inequalities in health: an assessment of the evidence', *Sociology of Health and Illness*, vol 9, pp 231-64.

Bourdieu, P. (1986) 'Forms of capital', in J.G. Richardson (ed) *Handbook of Theory and Research for the Sociology of Education*, New York, NY: Greenwood Press.

Bourdieu, P., Ferguson, P.P., Emanuel, S. et al (1999) *The Weight of the World: Social Suffering in Contemporary Society*, Cambridge: Polity Press.

Boyle, P., Curtis, S., Graham, E. and Moore, E. (2004) (eds) *The Geography of Health Inequalities in the Developed World*, Aldershot: Ashgate.

Cattell, V. (2001) 'Poor people, poor places and poor health: the mediating role of social networks and social capital', *Social Science and Medicine*, vol 52, pp 1501-16.

Chief Medical Officer (2003) *Health in Wales: Chief Medical Officer's Report, 2001/2002*, Cardiff: Welsh Assembly Government.

Coalfields Task Force (1998) *Making the Difference: A New Start for England's Coalfield Communities*, London: Department for Environment, Transport and the Regions.

Dahlgren, G. and Whitehead, M. (1991) *Policies and Strategies to Promote Social Equity in Health*, Stockholm: Institute of Futures Studies

Davey Smith, G. and Kuh, D. (1997) 'Does early nutrition affect later health? Views from the 1930s and 1980s', in D.F. Smith (ed) *Nutrition in Britain: Science, Scientists and Politics in the Twentieth Century*, London: Routledge, pp 214-37.

Davey Smith, G., Blane, D. and Bartley, M. (1994) 'Explanations for socio-economic differences in mortality: evidence from Britain and elsewhere', *European Journal of Public Health*, vol 4, pp 131-44.

DH (Department of Health) (1999) *Saving Lives: Our Healthier Nation*, London: DH.

DHSS (Department of Health and Social Security) (1980) *Inequalities in Health: Report of a Working Group* (the Black Report), London: DHSS.

Elliott, E. and Williams, G. (2003) 'Developing a civic intelligence: local involvement in health impact assessment', *Environmental Impact Assessment Review*, vol 24, pp 231-43.

Fairbrother, P. and Morgan, K. (eds) (2001) *Steel Communities Study*, Cardiff: Regeneration Institute, Cardiff University.

Frohlich, K., Corin, E. and Potvin, L. (2001) 'A theoretical proposal for the relationship between context and disease', *Sociology of Health and Illness*, vol 23, pp 776-97.

Gordon, D. et al (2001) *Wales NHS Resource Allocation Review: Independent Report of the Research Team*, Cardiff: Welsh Assembly Government.

Graham, H. (2001) 'The challenge of health inequalities', in H. Graham (ed) *Understanding Health Inequalities*, Buckingham: Open University Press.

Graham, H. (2004) 'Tackling health inequalities in England: remedying health disadvantages, narrowing gaps or reducing health gradients', *Journal of Social Policy*, vol 33, pp 115-31.

Hart, J.T. (1971) 'The inverse care law', *Lancet*, vol 1, no 7696, pp 405-12.

Higgs, G., Senior, M.L. and Williams, H. (1998) 'Spatial and temporal variation of mortality and deprivation 1: widening health inequalities', *Environment and Planning A*, 30, pp 1661-82.

Hunter, D. (2003) *Public Health Policy*, Cambridge: Polity Press.

Ingold, T. (2000) *The Perception of the Environment: Essays in Livelihood, Dwelling and Skill*, London: Routledge.

Joshi, H., Wiggins, R., Bartley, M., Mitchell, R., Gleave, S. and Lynch, K. (2001) 'Putting health inequalities on the map: does where you live matter, and why?', in H. Graham (ed) *Understanding Health Inequalities*, Buckingham: Open University Press, pp 143-55.

Judge, K. and Bauld, L. (2005) 'Conclusion', in M. Barnes, L. Bauld, M. Benzeval, K. Judge, M. Mackenzie and H. Sullivan (eds) *Health Action Zones: Partnerships for Health Equity*, London: Routledge.

Macintyre, S. (1997) 'The Black Report and beyond: what are the issues?', *Social Science and Medicine*, vol 44, pp 723-45.

Macintyre, S. (2000) 'Modernising the NHS: prevention and the reduction of inequalities', *British Medical Journal*, vol 320, pp 1399-400.

Marmot, M. (1998) 'The magnitude of social inequalities in coronary heart disease', in I. Sharp (ed) *Social Inequalities in Coronary Heart Disease* London: The Stationery Office.

Marmot, M. and Shipley, M. (1996) 'Do socioeconomic differences in mortality persist after retirement? 25 year follow-up of civil servants from the Whitehall Study', *British Medical Journal*, vol 313, pp 1177-80.

McKeown, T. (1979) *The Role of Medicine: Dream, Mirage or Nemesis*, Oxford: Oxford University Press.

National Assembly for Wales (1999) *Welsh Health Survey 1998*, Cardiff: National Assembly for Wales.

National Assembly for Wales (2001a) *NHS Resource Allocation Review. Targeting Poor Health: Professor Townsend's Report of the Welsh Assembly's National Steering Group on the Allocation of NHS Resources*, Cardiff: Welsh Assembly Government.

National Assembly for Wales (2001b) *Improving Health in Wales: A Plan for the NHS with its Partners*, Cardiff: National Assembly for Wales

National Assembly for Wales (2003) *A Statistical Focus on Disability and Long-Term Illness in Wales*, Cardiff: Statistical Directorate, National Assembly for Wales.

ONS (Office for National Statistics) (2005) *Life Expectancy at Birth by Health and Local Authorities in the United Kingdom, 1991–1993 to 2002–2004*, London: ONS.

Popay, J., Williams, G., Thomas, C. and Gatrell, A, (1998) 'Theorising inequalities in health: the place of lay knowledge', in M. Bartley, D. Blane and G. Davey Smith (eds) *The Sociology of Health Inequalities*, Oxford: Blackwell, pp 59-84.

Popay, J., Thomas, C., Williams, G., Bennett, S., Gatrell, A., and Bostock, L. (2003a) 'A proper place to live: health inequalities, agency and the normative dimensions of space', *Social Science and Medicine*, vol 57, pp 55-69.

Popay J., Bennett, S., Thomas, C., Williams, G., Gatrell, A. and Bostock, L. (2003b) 'Beyond "beer, fags, egg and chips"? Exploring lay understandings of social inequalities in health', *Sociology of Health and Illness*, vol 25, pp 1-15.

Pope, R. (1998) *Building Jerusalem: Nonconformity, Labour and the Social Question in Wales, 1906–1939*, Cardiff: University of Wales Press.

Power, C., Matthews, S. and Manor, O. (1996) 'Inequalities in self-rated health in the 1958 birth cohort: life time social circumstances or social mobility?', *British Medical Journal*, vol 313, pp 449-53.

Shaw, M., Dorling, D., Gordon, D. and Davey Smith, G. (1999) *The Widening Gap: Health Inequalities and Policy in Britain*, Bristol: Policy Press.

Shaw, M., Davey Smith, G. and Dorling, D. (2007) 'Health inequalities and New Labour: how the promises compare with real progress', *British Medical Journal*, vol 330, pp 1016-21.

Shim, J.K. (2002) 'Understanding the routinised inclusion of race, socio-economic status and sex in epidemiology: the utility of concepts from technoscience studies', *Sociology of Health and Illness*, vol 24, pp 129-50.

Smith, D. (1993) *Aneurin Bevan and the World of South Wales*, Cardiff: University of Wales Press.

Smith, D. (1999) *Wales: A Question for History*, Bridgend: Seren.

Smith, S. and Easterlow, D. (2005) 'The strange geography of health inequalities', *Transactions of the Institute of British Geographers*, vol 30, pp 173-90.

Townsend, P., Davidson N. and Whitehead, M. (1988) *Inequalities in Health: The Black Report and the Health Divide*, Harmondsworth: Penguin.

Vågerö, D. and Illsley, R. (1995) 'Explaining health inequalities: beyond Black and Barker', *European Sociological Review*, vol 11, pp 219-41.

Wanless, D. (2004) *Securing Good Health for the Whole Population: Final Report* (the Wanless Report), London: HM Treasury.

Welsh Assembly Government (2002) *Well Being in Wales: A Consultation Document*, Cardiff: Welsh Assembly Government.

Welsh Assembly Government (2003) *The Review of Health and Social Care in Wales: The Report of the Project Team Advised by Derek Wanless*, Cardiff: Welsh Assembly Government.

Welsh Assembly Government (2006) *Communities First: A 2001 Baseline*, Cardiff: Statistical Policy Unit, Welsh Assembly Government.

Welsh Office (1998) *Better Health – Better Wales*, Cm 3922, Cardiff: The Stationery Office.

Whitehead, M. (1987) *The Health Divide: Inequalities in Health in the 1980s*, London: Health Education Council.

Wilkinson, R. (1976) 'Dear Mr Ennals', *New Society*, 16 December, pp 567-8.

Wilkinson, R. (1996) *Unhealthy Societies: The Afflictions of Inequality*, London: Routledge.

Wilkinson, R. (2005) *The Impact of Inequality: How to Make Sick Societies Healthier*, London: Routledge.

Williams, C. (1998) *Capitalism, Community and Conflict: The South Wales Coalfield, 1898-1947*, Cardiff: University of Wales Press.

Williams, G.H. (2003) 'The determinants of health: structure, context and agency', *Sociology of Health and Illness*, vol 25, pp 131-54.

Williams, G.H. (2006) 'History is what you live: understanding health inequalities in Wales', in P. Michael and C. Webster (eds) *Health and Society in Twentieth Century Wales*, Cardiff: University of Wales Press.

TWO

'Policy experiments': policy making, implementation and learning

Steve Cropper and Mark Goodwin

Introduction

There is an enduring interest in the ways in which public policy is formed, communicated and embedded into public (and private) life. We might expect that, where policy directly addresses community and individual well-being and health, there would be intense debate about the content of policy, especially as its implications for the distribution of responsibility, authority and action become clear. Given this, the design or, perhaps, the unfolding of the policy process is also a matter of some importance. A classic 1960s study of community politics asked: 'Who governs?' (Dahl, 1963). In commenting on Dahl's study, Saunders (1979) noted that the question of legitimacy is central to the design of what we now increasingly refer to as 'the system of governance'. This idea of governance gives less privilege to the 'centre of government' from which policy is determined and issued, but rather sees policy as emerging from a series of influences and negotiations, openings and resistances that interested parties might seek and take as legitimate opportunities to engage or not. The 'opportunity structure', that is, the distribution of different forms of access to power, is changing, the intention being to broaden involvement in policy making at all levels of government and indeed of relevant agency. The debate about health inequalities, and where responsibility for action on health inequalities rests, continues. Despite hints of movement towards government and the corporation, with their greater institutional leverage on environments, the distribution of wealth and lifestyle products, there has equally been emphasis on individual choice (of lifestyle) – most clearly signalled in the English public health White Paper *Choosing Health* (DH, 2004). The question, then, is how policy comes into being and is sustained, or otherwise; this may be of most interest in the range of practices it seeks to influence, but policy may colonise practices it did not seek to affect and it may fail to touch practices of central concern.

In this chapter, then, we consider the nature of public policy and the ways in which policy is made, and we examine attempts to improve policy making and its effectiveness, in particular against a challenging agenda of revitalisation of welfare and public service. Against the emergence of health and health inequalities as public policy concerns set out by Gareth Williams in Chapter One, the following chapter then discusses how the Sustainable Health Action Research Programme (SHARP) could be established as both an action and a research (or policy learning[a]) programme.

Public policy: distinctions and debates

There are a number of excellent general accounts of public policy making and policy implementation that rehearse the debates about policy and policy making. Reports of research into agenda setting (Kingdon, 2003), policy implementation (Pressman and Wildavsky, 1974; Bardach, 1977; Barrett and Fudge, 1981) and policy networks (Rhodes, 1997) have helped to unravel the making and delivery of public policy, suggesting alternatives to a rather tidy, normative account of the way policy *should* rationally be made. It has always been clear that in democratic societies there is political contest over the extent of governmental responsibility and power, and about the substantive direction and form of policy. But, in addition, there have been attempts to assert a strong scientific rationality as a basis for policy, and to maintain an administrative orderliness, control and predictability in implementation. Both searches for order continue, the first, for example, in the investments in evidence-based policy making (Davies et al, 2000; Sanderson, 2002; Nutley et al, 2007) and the latter in various performance management regimes. But there has been an accumulation of evidence that the course of public policy seldom follows simple or idealised models of the policy-making and implementation process. It is not so much that public policy issues are nowadays more complex, although that *might* be a legitimate claim not least in the area of health inequalities, but rather that understanding of the policy process has been enriched.

Accounts of the change in British public policy and in the character of policy making following New Labour's election to power in 1997 after 17 years of a Conservative administration have perhaps exaggerated these general tendencies. The accounts point up change to the substance, or content, of policy, in particular the return to strong commitments to public and collective welfare provision, albeit a version strongly influenced by the politics and policies of the 1980s and 1990s (eg Paton, 2006). But Newman (2001) and Barnes and colleagues (2005) note that alongside New Labour's determination to transform public policy and public services, there was also a commitment to improve the processes of government policy making.

The distinction drawn between the *content* of policy and the *processes* through which policy is determined is an analytical one. The former – the content of policy – refers to the substantive character of policy (the terms in which it specifies problems – economic competitiveness, social exclusion, urban regeneration, rural development, health inequalities, and so forth) as societal priorities, and the direction, nature and responsibilities attaching to a response. As the discussion in Chapter One has suggested, policy analysis would be interested in the coherence and the moral, scientific and practical force of the policy argument, and the extent to which the measures specified can be judged to lead specifically and effectively to the policy ends. The latter – policy processes – concern the forms of deliberation that lead to policy. Here, then, we find the debates about how policy is made and how it should be made, and more generally, as we will see below, about the way in which the policy process is conceived – should we think of policy design as separate from policy implementation, for example?

The distinction between content and process reflects Herbert Simon's separation of substantive and procedural rationalities (Simon, 1982). A focus on the variety of forms of rationality is helpful in pointing to different criteria against which to judge policy and the bases on which policy and action are founded. Was the policy valid – did the measures that made up the action programme make progress toward the policy objectives? Or was the process by which it was made of high quality – inclusive, informed and testing? Both are reasonable questions in retrospect, but at the time of making the decision, the decisive question (and response to challenge) is often about the adequacy of process. The previous chapter examined the substantive case for action, and particular types of action, on health inequalities: here, the focus is on process as the primary concern.

It is also useful to set out the terms in which we describe and seek to explain policy processes. Political and professional leadership, the processes of policy making and implementation, the institutions – political, economic and social – within which policy is made and delivered, and the trends within broader political economy are all candidates. Hudson and Lowe (2004), for example, talk of micro, meso and macro levels of analysis, respectively. At the *micro* level, our attention is drawn to the contributions that individuals and groups make to policy as it is formed and takes effect, and to processes that involve interactions between individuals and groups – as policy analysts and advocates – over the strength or relevance of evidence, and in making judgements and decisions that affect the nature of policy. At the *meso* level, we are concerned with the way in which those individual contributions are shaped by precedents and rules, norms, set beliefs, and the way organisations are structured and behave – institutional features that exert powerful influences over what can be done. As Hudson and Lowe (2004, p 11) suggest: 'Meso-level analysis is thus characterised by two distinct features: the use of middle range theory to explain the policy process from the moment a social problem is identified – following the various stages of design and implementation – and the emphasis on the cultural/historical explanation for how the welfare states of different countries differ.'

Although there is a developing debate about tendencies to convergence or divergence in the welfare policies and systems of delivery of states, not only globally, but also within the UK (for health inequalities specifically, see, for example, the introduction to Graham, 2004), this takes us towards the macro level of analysis and to the forces that shape policy in the broadest sense. Hudson and Lowe (2004) include globalisation and big trends in the political economy, in technology and social patterning (see also Ozga, 2005). In terms of the process of policy making at the macro level, Greer (2004), for example, examines and explains divergences in health policy, not by reference to differing character of health problems in the four nations of the UK, but rather in terms of devolution, 'territorial politics' and the search for politically distinctive programmes of welfare development. But equally, we can see that health inequalities have become a policy issue of importance across the UK, and indeed, elsewhere (see, for example, Graham, 2004; Freeman, 2006). The spread of a policy issue and of policy responses, internationally, is equally an institutional effect (Marmor et al, 2005).

Although questions of the mechanisms of policy differentiation, convergence and transfer are interesting and important, the focus of the account in this book, as the analysis in Chapter One has signalled, is at the micro and meso levels and in trying to unpick the complexities of policy making and innovation. Specifically, we are concerned with mapping out processes by which a policy direction can be tested, made sense of, elaborated and closely connected to action. We are also concerned with the learning that emanates from such processes.

First, however, we go back a step and ask what is meant by the term 'policy'.

New Labour, public policy and wicked problems

In her analysis of New Labour's reform of governance, Janet Newman (2001) noted that the attempt to redress what New Labour saw as policy failure in the UK was bound up with a commitment to tackle what Horst Rittel and Marvin Webber (1973) termed 'wicked problems'. Although there was still a focus on traditional public policy and public services in New Labour's political programme (Tony Blair's articulation of 'education, education, education' is perhaps the most memorable example), a number of what became known as 'cross-cutting' issues became a central part of the incoming administration's distinctive approach to government and to policy. These issues included poverty and inequality, social exclusion and democratic renewal and each has been a key element of social and community policy since 1997.

A series of diagnostic documents (Cabinet Office, 1999a, 1999b), reviewed by Newman (2001, p 63), set out the requirements of policy making and delivery that would meet the challenge of the 'wicked problems' that had been neither on the agenda nor capable of being addressed using the policy levers favoured in the past decade and more. A subsequent discussion paper, *'Better Policy Design and Delivery'* also sought to provoke 'more rigorous thinking about delivery issues within Government' (PIU, 2001). It summarises the conventional theory of policy making and delivery as follows:

- Politicians identify a priority and the broad outlines of a solution....
- Policy-makers in Whitehall design a policy to put this into effect, assembling the right collection of tools: legislation, funding, incentives, new institutions, directives.
- The job of implementation is then handed over to a different group of staff; an agency or local government.
- ... the goal is (hopefully) achieved. (Performance and Innovation Unit, 2001, p 5)

It goes on to identify what would be required to ensure that policy follows this progression: directness in movement of policy along the process, clarity and specificity of policy prescription, clear accountabilities, and effective sanctions on each link in the chain to encourage or ensure performance. And the paper reflects on why such a model of the policy process, although normatively appealing and intellectually clear, may be inadequate as a basis for the design of policy governance. It concludes that a more refined methodology for policy making is required. We pick up four points the paper makes.

First, the paper draws a distinction between measures leading to the implementation of policy, the achievement of targets and the achievement of better outcomes: all form interconnected parts of a delivery chain. Although these may be coherent and aligned, equally they can be in tension. Excessive focus on change and on targets can lead to perverse effects – skewing or frustrating the range of action needed to achieve long-term outcomes. There is recognition, then, of the difficulty in understanding and of building into policy designs the complex chains of means that lead to the intended, long-term effects.

Second, and related, central control over the delivery chain is limited. The paper points out that limited central understanding of the variety that is found among practice settings may mean that policy design does not allow for that variety and this may lead to the local failure of policy. Other factors that complicate the delivery of policy are identified – difficulty in anticipating all the changes to systems that are required to enable policy delivery, and equally, the impact of changes on other policies. The paper recognises that implementation of policy occurs 'at the front line' through the actions of many professionals, 'street-level bureaucrats' (Lipsky, 1980). Translation of policy into practice, at minimum, will involve exercise of discretion in interpreting policy and adapting it to the particular case or to local settings.

Third, such an intelligent capacity for implementation is required because policy is seldom fully defined, or definitive. As the paper argues, '… in practice ideas are tested either in pilots … or prototypes and pathfinders where policies have to be rapidly adapted in the light of early experience. The more quickly policies are adapted in the light of experience, drawing lessons from the frontline, the more chance they have of succeeding' (PIU, 2001, p 7).

Finally, the paper points to the sheer intractability of the issues New Labour was seeking to address – many of the issues that policy has sought to address are likely to be affected only through sustained attention, the redistribution of significant resources, and extraordinary degrees of response to policy by the variety of stakeholders – from the individual to government itself. With cross-cutting issues, the task of 'joining up' policy responses has been significant. As Rittel and Webber (1973) pointed out, wicked problems are not just matters to do with technical competence; they also require institutional adjustment. It is in these terms that we can understand New Labour's preoccupation with partnership working and with new forms of democratic practice within public services.

Indeed, though it retains a sense of a privileged policy centre within which the primary responsibility for the gathering, analysis and determination of policy is located, the Performance and Innovation Unit's paper opens up the possibility of a more interactive policy process.[b] There have been two critiques of such a position. The first challenges the capacity of such a centre to undertake policy analysis and design, especially with the added complexities of participatory processes; the second asks whether policy can usefully be conceived in these terms at all and whether, instead, policy should be seen as emergent, formed and located in many locations, understandings and practices, and as effects that depend more on organisational behaviour than on the rightness of analysis. We explore this issue of organisation for policy making and policy learning below, in our discussion of governance, but consider, first, the challenges of problem analysis and policy design.

Policy design, complexities and policy stress

John Friend's (1977) paper on the dynamics of policy change asked how policy might be adapted and designed to make a positive contribution to public planning efforts, albeit given a 'realistic appreciation of the limits of policy influence within a complex "organisational ecology"' (p 45). He distinguishes policy (the general aspiration or position) from decisions (totally specific in terms of classifying situations and prescribing responses), arguing that while decisions are acts that 'once made pass into history' (p 40), policy is a forward-looking stance that forms part of the contexts in which future decisions will be made. It is 'part of the context', since other considerations come to bear in the act of decision, including other policies. Friend coins the term 'policy stress' to describe the manner in which policy statements start to decay and to become undermined by three types of change: change in the operating environment, responsiveness to stakeholder interests and the inherent complexity of problems. The second and third, in particular, may have a tendency 'to increase the degree of perceived incompatibility between one policy statement and another ...' (p 45). Friend argues that the design and adaptation of policy will be contested: some interests will seek greater specificity in the content and scope of application of policy; other interests may find it 'important to retain the freedom to negotiate over policy interpretation' (p 44).

We pick up two points from Friend's analysis, which are reflected in continuing debate about the design of policy. The first concerns his point about the complexity of problem structure and the degree to which policy seeks to define what to do, or merely to signal broad intent to act. As we have noted, New Labour's programme identified a set of interlinked social issues, each complex, each deeply rooted and enduring, and for each, the question is how best to catalyse and coordinate action that has demonstrable impact. The second concerns change in the operating environment. If policy is an attempt to support and shape decisions – that is, to help in responding to uncertainty about what to do – then policy itself will depend on a set of assumptions about the future operating environment and what the effects of policy would be. Both points take us to debates about evidence-based policy and practice (Davies et al, 2000) and the handling of uncertainty.

Graham (2004) notes that at least three meanings have become attached to the term health inequalities (see also the discussion in Chapter One), each with their own distinctive set of assumptions and action imperatives. 'Remedying the health disadvantage' of poor groups and communities requires attention to reduce absolute social disadvantage experienced by these groups – by action addressing the so-called wider determinants of health – 'poverty, poor housing, pollution, low educational standards, joblessness and low pay' (Graham, 2004, pp 119-20). This version points to links between public health policy and other elements of the welfare programme, including work to tackle social exclusion and, inter alia, to area-based measures. 'Narrowing health gaps' follows this same logic, but its targets are more challenging: rather than seeking absolute improvement in the health of the poorest groups and communities, narrowing the gap requires policy to realise a faster rate of improvement for these groups than for those with better health. Finally, reducing health gradients is not just about the differences between poorer and better-off groups, but about the systematic relationship between socioeconomic position and health: this requires a population-wide response.

As Graham (2004, pp 127-8) notes in conclusion:

> An important first step is clarity about goals ... what counts as a health inequality if they [researchers, policy makers, practitioners] are to inform, develop and deliver strategies which can contribute to greater equality in health.

Rationalist theories of policy making certainly reflect Graham's plea for clarity about ends. But uncertainty can also be a matter of ignorance about the causal mechanisms that policy might seek to trigger to bring about change. In wicked problems, the pathways may be circular – poverty leads to poor health, which in turn feeds back to continuing deprivation. They may also be diffuse and long. And it may be unclear which ways into the system of issues provide the most appropriate starting points or the most powerful levers. Petticrew and colleagues (2003), in exploring differences between researchers' and policy makers' appraisal of the evidence base to support choice of strategy to address inequalities in health, find that 'the type of evidence sought ... that is evidence on the means of addressing the social determinants of health inequalities – is sparse, and is often less accessible than clinical evidence....' (p 814) and that policy makers point 'to a need for stronger theoretical underpinnings ... to take account of plausible causal pathways....' (p 815). Uncertainty in policy design, then, may be a reflection of what O'Toole and Meier (2003) term programmatic uncertainty; specifically, that 'decision makers simply do not know enough (about the actions of others, the consequences of these, or even the consequences of their own choices) to select programme actions or elements that they will be sure will lead to desired outcomes' (p 100).

It is not goals, then, that are the sole subject of uncertainty or lack of agreement in policy making: choices are made about 'means' too, and these choices can fundamentally influence the character of policy. Indeed, if we take the findings of implementation studies (Barrett and Fudge, 1981; Allen, 2001), policy literally is formed and given substance as it is implemented. As Davies et al (2000) note:

> Practitioners do not merely implement policy decisions that have been decided elsewhere. Policy is influenced from the bottom up ... as well as practice being influenced from the top down.... The phrase policy making does not usually relate to a clearly defined event or to an explicit set of decisions. Policy tends to emerge and accrete rather than being the outcome of conscious deliberation.... (Davies et al, 2000, p 15)

Especially where the range of potential action responses to policy is wide, or distributed, the set of responses in practice may not be easy to anticipate, coordinate or control. Too specific a set of policy goals may restrict the range of response. So Baier and colleagues (1988) have argued that: 'Policy ambiguity allows different groups and individuals to support the same policy for different reasons, and with different expectations, including different expectations about the administrative consequences of the policy. Thus official policy is likely to be vague, contradictory or adopted without generally shared expectations about its meaning or implementation' (p 157).

Thompson's (2003) analysis of modes of decision making provides a way of considering these observations about policy making. His original concern was to understand how a 'dominant coalition' could carry and sustain the action programme of an organisation and there are clear parallels with the policy process and the politics of policy – the ways in which, as Klein (1989, pp 243-4) puts it, 'we perceive and define policy issues and our sense of what is possible and feasible'. On the first dimension, 'ends' or goals, placement of a policy issue in the category of 'certain' or 'uncertain' would imply that a consensus does or does not exist among the primary stakeholders about what would constitute a desirable outcome (or equally outcomes to be avoided). On the second dimension, 'means', similarly, there can be more or less certainty about what would work.

Drawing together these two sources of uncertainty (or indeed ambiguity) about ends and about means, respectively, led Thompson to distinguish between four types of context that we can see as describing the state of 'policy knowledge'. Tame problems are those that are understood and, within prevailing institutional frameworks, capable of an effective response. Wicked problems are those that are less well understood and inherently complex and for which there is likely to be a mismatch between the organisation required to address the problem and the current institutional framework. Table 2.1 indicates the four types of context in which policy might be located and (in italics) the types of policy-making and policy-learning responses that might best fit with each context.

Current policy-making norms call for an evidence-based approach. Although the pursuit of evidence to inform policy goals and action programmes may be desirable in principle, there are questions about

Table 2.1: Ends, means and uncertainty

		Ends	
		Certain	**Uncertain**
Means	**Certain**	Tame problems *Evidence-based policy making*	Political/leadership crisis *Policy/political debate*
	Uncertain	Wicked problems *Innovation, experiment and policy learning*	Wicked problems *Muddling through*

Source: Thompson (2003)

whether evidence-based policy making is the most appropriate response. Health inequalities policy may call for a partnership of responsible agencies; yet the institutional pressures remain strong to pursue core activities in relation to particular, sectoral, policy goals. For a policy such as health inequalities, the starting point may be to focus on an elaboration of possible actions to address inequalities, and since the policy goals themselves are weakly specified and asserted, to move between action (termed 'muddling through' by Lindblom (1959)) and deliberate, designed, processes of policy learning. Learning is in part about 'what works' and in part about what would make for an institutional capacity capable of delivering effective interventions.

Policy implementation: governance and organisation of the policy system

New Labour's policies have proved to be demanding on executive and administrative structures that remain highly departmentalised and disconnected, both at central government level and among local agencies. The task of 'joining up' has been central to the programme of cross-cutting issues and a range of measures – structural, exhortatory and mandatory – have been tried to repair what are perhaps inevitable failures of organisation. As Challis and colleagues (1988) have commented, in assessing an earlier attempt to improve coordination of social policy making in government: 'The implication … is that what is required is coordination between different policies, each of which is designed to meet one of an interlocking set of needs. The real problem of coordination is seen to lie at the interface between the major strands of social policy and the major service departments and agencies which enact them' (p 36). They go on to argue that:

> This is a wholly misleading picture and it is one which arises from the conceptualisation of policy as a coherent, relatively self-contained, complete and authoritative guide to future action…. In reality, policy processes are altogether more complex and messy. The conflicts and power struggles which determine the outcomes of social policy (as opposed to the content of statements of objectives which are merely inputs) are to be located throughout the government system and not only in 'the social policy departments'. (p 37)

Challis and colleagues' (1988) suggestion is to recognise the complexities of policy making and implementation. They point to Kingdon's (2003) idea of a 'policy primeval soup': in contrast to more classical accounts of power or bureaucratic politics, Kingdon characterises policy making as a disorderly, essentially random process of policy survival,

> ... in which specialists try out their ideas in a variety of ways ... proposals are floated, come into contact with one another, are revised and combined with one another, and floated again. But the proposals that survive to the status of serious consideration meet several criteria, including their technical feasibility, their fit with dominant values and the current national mood, their budgetary workability, and the political support or opposition they might meet. (Kingdon, 2003, pp 19-20)

The lack of attention to how policy could command authority, ownership and attention across traditional lines was the subject of comment in the evaluation of England's first comprehensive public health policy – *The Health of the Nation* (DH, 1998). Although New Labour has sought to spread authority on, and responsibility for, cross-cutting issues through policy coordinating centres, multiple ministerial signatures, duty of partnership, reform of local structures, and so forth, the conclusion that government's reliance on action along the traditional lines of authority led to weak responses from agencies with responsibility for wider determinants of health, notably in local authorities – education, housing, transport and so on – may still apply.

The task of joining up, then, is complex. Lateral connections in government, the vertical connections between central and local agents and the lateral connections between the various local agents all need to be aligned for 'policy windows to be opened' (Exworthy and Powell, 2004). Conflict between short- and long-term intentions, between one instruction and another, and between the priorities of one policy operator and another all point to a complex politics of implementation in the context of fragmented accountabilities. In addition to the complexities of organisational jurisdiction and priority, there are issues simply about learning to work in new ways and embedding these in routines (Schofield, 2004). Especially where local organisations are newly formed and complex themselves – Children's Trusts, local health alliances, health and wellbeing partnerships and so on – the task of establishing organisational presence and of creating routines in the face of those of long-standing organisations is a challenge. Small wonder, with such potential for policy stress, then, that implementation studies including those by Bardach (1977) and Barratt and Fudge (1981) have observed no straightforward translation from policy to practice. Since

Pressman and Wildavsky's classic study of 'the implementation gap', the expectation that centrally written policy should be seen as what Elmore (1979) in his classic paper terms 'the determinant influence over what happens in the implementation process', whether or not it is explicit, clear, or well-defined, has been challenged. Nor is there much 'useful' research (O'Toole, 1986, 2004), other than some rather straightforward suggestions. As Elmore (1979, p 601) argues: 'Better policies would result, we are told, if policy makers would think about whether their decisions could be implemented before they settle on a course of action'. His 'backward mapping' method traces back from 'the last possible stage, the point at which administrative actions intersect private choices. It begins not with a statement of intent but with a statement of the specific behaviour at the lowest level of the implementation process' (p 604).

The design of policy may therefore involve that element of programmatic uncertainty, termed implementation uncertainty by O'Toole and Meier (2003, p 101) and which they suggest is 'associated with the challenge of assembling predictable and cooperative action among implementers themselves. This issue is at the heart of public management – coordinating people and other resources to carry out policies'.

Newman (2001) suggests that the New Labour government moved from a position that saw the public sector as a *target of reform* (essentially the position taken by the preceding conservative government) to one in which sub-central government was viewed as a *mechanism and agent of social change*. The emphasis shifted from radical institutional change, including the introduction of a whole range of market-like mechanisms into the public services to a view of the public sector as a crucial means of delivering social policy. Newman suggests that the style of policy making and policy implementation moved similarly: from one that was 'top-down, mandatory and prescriptive' to a more interactive, inclusive approach to policy making as part of a new style of governance. Indeed, Exworthy and colleagues (2002) note:

> Health inequalities may indeed be a national priority but it does not follow that this will necessarily precipitate local action. Issues may thus need to appear both on national and local agendas before implementation occurs. (Exworthy et al, 2002, p 80)

This is consistent with more recent thinking about systems of governance that reflect change in the role of public agencies from simply direct providers of services to commissioners, contractors, enablers and leaders.

Where public services had once been the sole province of central and local government, the new systems of governance involve a wide range of agencies drawn from the public, private and voluntary sectors. These still include the institutions of elected government, but also involve a range of non-elected organisations of the state, as well as institutional and individual actors from outside the formal political arena, such as voluntary organisations, private businesses and corporations and supra-national institutions such as the European Union. Reflecting these changes, the term 'governance' is thus used to refer to 'the development of governing styles in which boundaries between and within public and private sectors have become blurred' (Stoker, 1998, p 17).

As a consequence, the range of agencies and organisations involved in the production of policy as effect or outcome in cross-cutting issues is bewildering, the degree of interest varies almost as much and the degree of control or influence that any single actor has is equally limited – although many now argue that local and central government still play a significant role in funding, coordinating and auditing these new governance networks (see Jessop, 2002). Since Rhodes' (1997) early and influential account of governance as a means of depicting this full range of responsible and engaged participants and active stakeholders in a fragmented polity, the idea has received significant attention (Newman, 2001, 2005; Kjaer, 2004). Rhodes characterised governance as a '*new* process of governing; or a *changed* condition of ordered rule' (1997, pp 52-3, emphasis in original), thus drawing our attention to the ways in which governmental and non-governmental organisations work together, and to the ways in which political power is distributed, both internal and external to the state. Hence we are also drawn to examine the articulation of governance networks – the tangled web of issue networks, policy networks and policy fields as a way of analysing the spread of interests and influences on policy.

We can look, for an example, at obesity in the child population, recently the subject of a report from the National Audit Office, Audit Commission and Healthcare Commission (2006b). The question identified is how concerted action can be established across public and private domains. A newspaper front page headline (*The Times*, 2006) reads 'Children grow fatter as the experts dither'; the diagram in the report from the National Audit Office, Audit Commission and Healthcare Commission (2006, p 30) reveals a range of responsible agencies: five government departments, a range of national government agencies and inspectorates, and local agencies and services are implicated. All 26 boxes indicated are public service organisations, but of course, private sector organisations, voluntary and community organisations and families also have a great influence on whether or not this is a problem fuelled or addressed. There is little definitive evidence about what to do to address the problem – the report talks of a 'complex suite of programmes' and notes that some 20 interventions are set out in the government's draft plan. It concludes that the overriding problem is one of organisation (National Audit Office, Audit Commission and Healthcare Commission, 2006, p 28).

The idea of governance implies a less bureaucratic mode of organisation than the traditional sense of the transmission of policy through layers of (lesser) authority – from principal to implementing agent – down the line of central to local government, political body to executive and administrative bodies, to delivery at the front line. But for cross-cutting issues, the task is to move from negotiations, central to local, in which instruction and accountability are structured by established 'silos' to freer networks of engagement. As Exworthy and Powell (2004, p 266) note, 'policy ownership is important. All stakeholders must believe that it is 'their problem' and they must have a role to play in the partnership, with solutions within their control'.

And yet, experience with public health policy suggests that this is easily undermined (DH, 1998). In recognition of this need to draw the range of interests into cross-cutting policy domains, the systems of rules and organisation through which policy is structured and mediated (Kjaer, 2004) are being stretched and changed. The idea of 'interactive governance' for example, reflects and prescribes a negotiative or deliberative process (Amin and Hausner, 1997). Finally, use of the terms 'participative governance' (Newman, 2005) and 'democratic governance' (Skelcher, 2005; Sterling, 2005) emphasises a more inclusive process to which service users, citizens and publics can gain access. Both recognise the range of interests in policy and the legitimacy that 'opening up the policy process' can accord, even if in the process there are challenges to established elements of the governance system. For example, the encouragement of participation, lay representation and other forms of direct democracy in policy making may be seen as a challenge to well-understood forms of democratic representation (Stoker, 1998; Newman, 2005; Sterling, 2005). This is important, both because it acknowledges the need to reconstruct a hollowed-out public sphere and because in the context of 'wicked problems' various forms of 'lay knowledge', 'civic intelligence' or 'civic epistemology' will need to enter policy deliberations alongside expert-generated evidence (Elliott and Williams, 2003; Jasanoff, 2005). In Wales, the Beecham Report on citizen-centred services has pressed exactly this case (Welsh Assembly Government, 2006).

Newman's (2001) analysis and anticipation of the design of governance systems suggests that the move to change the systems, culture and style of policy making would be full of tensions and competing draws. Responses to different interests and ideologies will add elements to designs and reforms of governance arrangements that take systems in different directions. Calls for stronger accountability will tend to lead towards risk aversion, managerial control through 'plan and audit', and the political concentration of power as the overriding governance principles. Conversely, pressures for responsiveness are likely to shift design towards forms of 'open systems' governance that emphasise innovation, policy experimentation, a greater distribution of power and responsibility, and learning.

In the final section, we turn to consider this last mode of governance and ask how policy systems have sought to learn to design and deliver effective policy.

Policy learning

The relationships between government and the wider set of policy actors include attempts to shape and reshape both formal and informal commitments through the way in which policy is understood. Hood (1983) distinguishes between effectors and detectors among the tools of government. 'Policy' as a 'token of authority' that seeks to determine or to guide the future decisions and actions of others is only one of the range of elements that might make for a package of governmental intervention. Other effector tools include informational, financial and organisational tools, each of which can provide further specificity or force to the direction of policy. But Hood also identifies a range of tools for *detection* that bring information back to government – as Hood notes, 'a government without detectors cannot govern at all' (1983, p 112).

Thompson's (2003) typology of responses to decision contexts, set out above, suggests different approaches to policy learning. In particular, where there is agreement about policy ends but uncertainty about what to do (what to do for the best, and how to avoid the worst), we would expect to see an investment in exploratory action – limited application of effectors with evaluation (or strengthened 'detection' in Hood's terms). Indeed, as well as investing heavily in mechanisms for the development of a more evidence-based policy and practice and looking elsewhere for policy lessons, New Labour committed to

... learning from experience. Government should regard policy making as a continuous learning process, not as a series of one-off initiatives. We will improve our use of evidence and research so that we understand better the problems we are trying to address. We must make use of more pilot schemes to encourage innovations and test whether they work. We will ensure that all policies and programmes are clearly specified and evaluated, and the lessons of success and failure communicated and acted on. Feedback from those who implement and deliver policies and services is essential. (Cabinet Office, 1999a, cited in Newman, 2001, p 63)

As with policy making and implementation, the dominant sense of learning in public policy and action draws on a systems view of the world (Ozga, 2005; Freeman, 2006); in this view, feedback about performance or about the feasibility of proposals designed to enact policy would constitute policy learning. Yet, performance management systems are limited to what Argyris and Schon (1978) termed 'single loop learning': against a set of given indicators, standard returns can identify quickly outliers in those terms, but they are not intended to raise questions quickly about the terms in which performance is, itself, defined. That would require the more reflexive, self-critical forms of learning that would change the governing variables themselves – what Argyris and Schon (1978) call 'double-loop learning' and 'deutero learning'. All forms of learning are required for the governance of public policy programmes, but the emphasis has tended to be on forms of accountability in which tightness of plans and performance against expectation, whether against benchmarks, standards and targets set or proposed, take precedence over learning and adjustment. In other words, the predominant focus is on the single loop.

The field of evaluation studies, with its strong presence in public policy and programmes of intervention has offered new ways of thinking about complex policy and delivery (see Chapter Seven). First, the very idea of policy as a theory (Majone, 1980) has become a central idea in theories of evaluation of policy (Weiss, 1995; Pawson and Tilley, 1997; Barnes et al, 2005). As Sanderson (2002, p 19) notes:

... we need to recognise that policies are essentially 'conjectures' based upon the best possible evidence. In most areas of economic and social policy this evidence will provide only partial confidence that policy interventions

> will work as intended. Consequently, such policy conjectures
> must be subject to rigorous testing.

While this suggests a tentativeness about policy that perhaps sits uncomfortably with the level of conviction required in the politics of policy and accountability, nevertheless, piloting and testing of new policy proposals has been a common approach in public policy. Sanderson (2002) points to areas such as crime prevention, employment and welfare policy, health education and local government, where a range of initiatives has been subject to comprehensive evaluation, both for impact and for the process of implementation. Pilots may start as interventions 'targeted' on the most needy communities, justified on the grounds of justice before they become a part of universal provision (for example, Sure Start Children's Centres), or they may be means of drawing learning from the 'trailblazers'. Sanderson draws attention to a distinction between piloting and 'prototyping', the latter useful when the concern is to assess *how* rather than *whether* a policy or action works. Yet, he suggests, the evaluations cannot easily provide the sort of evidence to respond to the two questions policy makers pose – 'Does it work?' and 'How can we best make it work?'. Innovative programmes need to stabilise before they can be evaluated fairly and yet the political process generally requires both constant change and quick answers. Barnes and colleagues (2005) bemoan the early closure of the Health Action Zones experiment and evaluation; and the national evaluation of Sure Start has similarly closed early and may be unable to reach a strong conclusion about the effectiveness of its programme or the interventions that made it up. Increasingly, evaluations focus on processes of implementation first, aiming to articulate the theories of practice that emerge as broad directions and resources are translated into action and specific packages of investment. Yet, as the Health Action Zones evaluation concluded, these theories of change, too, can be hard to codify (Barnes et al, 2005).

In sum, the relationship between evidence and policy remains unpredictable (Nutley et al, 2007). Evidence to define which means to select for a new, or complex, policy is likely to be fragmentary; and the learning about policy experiments may be undermined by policy ambiguity and complexity, by political rather than scientific timeframes, by the dominant investment in single-loop rather than double-loop capacities, and by difficulties in translating findings back from the 'field' to policy makers and their deliberations. Weiss (1991) highlighted three types of material that policy makers would see as relevant and might use to inform policy: facts, ideas and arguments. But she has also suggested that evaluation and social science research seldom influence policy very directly. Rather, it seem likely that there is a more diffuse process of 'enlightenment' in which knowledge accretes to form broad movements in policy thinking. Although research and evaluation are important means of learning from policy experiments, alternative forms of policy learning are also being pursued, in part to return experience from the front line to policy makers, but also to spread experience and energy for change. Professional networks and collaboratives, with government-sponsored brokers, seek to draw together thoughtful, experienced practitioners and to share wisdom about 'best practice' or indeed what policy might mean for action. Such forms of 'advice giving' may draw more on what Rein (1976, p 261) calls 'stories' that

> … may take the form of supplying supporting evidence for what the policy makers want to do, or reassurance. More often, the essential role of advice is to supply contradictory evidence, pointing to the limits of the policy maker's ideas or programmes, or speculating and, better still, supplying evidence, about the possibility of unanticipated consequences.

Importantly, stories make sense locally as well as at more aggregate levels of policy making (see also Freeman, 2006). They are recognisable for their basis in lived experience as well as for the arguments and morals they carry (see Sims, 1999) and so they may not only be more 'democratic' but also more directly generative of action than quantitative evidence (Schon, 1979; Crossa, 2005). The recognition that policy is made and remade in many places – through action and inaction, negotiation, acceptance and denial, as much as through evidence – means that the forms of evidence that connect, the timing of evidence use and the media through which evidence is communicated are all as varied as the audiences to which it is addressed and the locales into which it is placed. Where there is authority, or discretion, evidence is part, but only a part, of a package of materials that are used to construct and refine policy and its counterparts in action.

Conclusion

Policy has been seen, conventionally, as a responsibility, right and good of government, and the dominant conception of implementation has been as a straightforward enactment of policy instruction by agents of government. But when control over knowledge and the possibility of action is seen as widely distributed, and as the complexities of social issues, policy design and 'governance' are recognised, it is clear that policy requires legitimacy other than governmental authority if it is to be carried through. That much is clear from 40 years of research into policy and implementation. There has been a search for sources of legitimacy both in the substance and the processes of policy making. In particular, the recent movement into evidence-based policy making seeks to address the requirements of substantive rationality and may also now represent a part of due procedure. Consultations with the widest range of stakeholders addresses the demands of procedural rationality primarily, but may also strengthen the substantive base of policy, and this more interactive style of policy making has become a part of a more democratic conception of 'delivery'. For complex policy issues where the framing, specification and ownership of action remain unclear, policy learning and experimentation, shared among a range of stakeholders, may provide a platform for more effective immediate action and for wider and more sustained change.

The range of experiments and local innovation that have been provoked in response to policy reflects an awareness that a narrow base of scientific evidence is seldom sufficient to support policy and that policy emerges over time from the interaction between broad direction and the detail of local action. The design of deliberate experiments to examine the feasibility or worth of measures to enact policy is not unusual, but the choice of an idea for organising policy translation is rare. Chapter One set out the emergence of arguments for a policy on health inequalities and suggested that it may be appropriate to leave the choice of means open to local discretion – so that the particularities of place and the resources available within a community could influence the form change would take. It is to the specification of an experiment in action (and research) to address health inequalities at the community level that we turn in Chapter Three.

Notes

[a] Policy learning has an established meaning that relates to the transfer of policy from one institutional context to another – usually across national borders (for example, Marmor et al, 2005). Here, the term is used to denote a reflexive approach to policy making in which learning about the feasibility, appropriateness and effectiveness of policy and the mechanisms that effect policy is actively sought.

[b] There is continuing attention to policy making in government departments addressing both substantive and procedural rationalities and, not surprisingly,

a strongly 'centred' view of the policy process – see for example, the Department of Health's policy collaborative established in 2003 (www.dh.gov. uk/en/Publicationsandstatistics/Lettersandcirculars/Dearcolleagueletters/ DH_4006367) and its statement on 'making policy' (www.dh.gov.uk/en/ Aboutus/HowDHworks/Policydevelopment/DH_410600, as modified 1 March 2007).

References

Allen, C. (2001) 'They just don't live and breathe it like we do... Policy intentions and practice dilemmas in modern social policy and implementation networks', *Policy Studies*, vol 22, pp 149-66.

Amin, A. and Hausner, J. (1997) *Beyond Market and Hierarchy: Interactive Governance and Social Complexity*, Cheltenham: Edward Elgar.

Argyris, C. and Schon, D.A. (1978) *Organizational Learning: A Theory of Action Perspective*, Reading, MA: Addison-Wesley.

Baier, V.E., March, J.G. and Saetren, H. (1988) 'Implementation and ambiguity', in J.G. March (ed) *Decisions and Organizations*, Oxford/ New York, NY: Basil Blackwell, pp 150-64.

Bardach, E. (1977) *The Implementation Game: What Happens after a Bill becomes a Law*, Cambridge, MA: MIT Press.

Barnes, M., Bauld, L., Benzeval, M., Judge, K., Mackenzie, M. and Sullivan, H. (2005) *Health Action Zones: Partnerships for Health Equity*, London: Routledge.

Barrett, S. (2004) 'Implementation studies: time for a revival? Personal reflections on 20 years of implementation studies', *Public Administration*, vol 82, pp 249-62.

Barrett, S. and Fudge, C. (eds) (1981) *Policy and Action*, London: Methuen.

Cabinet Office (1999a) *Modernising Government*, Cm 4310, London: The Stationery Office.

Cabinet Office (1999b) *Professional Policy Making in the 21st Century*, London: Cabinet Office.

Challis, L., Fuller, S., Henwood, M., Klein, R., Plowden, W., Webb, A., Whittingham, P. and Wistow, G. (1988) *Joint Approaches to Social Policy. Rationality and Practice*, Cambridge: Cambridge University Press.

Crossa, V. (2005) 'Converting the "small stories" into "big" ones: a response to Susan Smith's "States, markets and an ethic of care"', *Political Geography*, vol 24, pp 29-34.

Dahl, R. (1963) *Who Governs?*, New Haven, CT: Yale University Press.

Davies, H.T.O., Nutley, S. and Smith, P.C. (2000) *What Works: Evidence-based Policy and Practice in Public Services*, Bristol: The Policy Press.

DH (Department of Health) (1998) *The Health of the Nation: A Policy Assessed*, London: The Stationery Office.

DH (2004) *Choosing Health: Making Healthy Choices Easier*, Cm 6374, London: The Stationery Office.

Elliott, E. and Williams, G. (2003) 'Developing a civic intelligence: local involvement in health impact assessment', *Environmental Impact Assessment Review*, vol 24, pp 231-43.

Elmore, R. (1979) 'Backward mapping: implementation research and policy decisions', *Political Science Quarterly*, vol 94, pp 601-21.

Exworthy, M. and Powell, M. (2004) 'Big windows and little windows: implementation in the "congested state"', *Public Administration*, vol 82, pp 263-81.

Exworthy, M., Berney, L. and Powell, M. (2002) 'How great expectations in Westminster may be dashed locally: the local implementation of national policy on health inequalities', *Policy and Politics*, vol 30, pp 79-96.

Freeman, R. (2006) 'The work the document does: research, policy and equity in health', *Journal of Health Politics, Policy and Law*, vol 31, pp 51-70.

Friend, J.K. (1977) 'The dynamics of policy change', *Long Range Planning*, vol 10, pp 40-7.

Graham, H. (2004) 'Tackling inequalities in health in England: remedying health disadvantages, narrowing health gaps or reducing health gradients', *Journal of Social Policy*, vol 33, pp 115-31.

Greer, S. (2004) *Territorial Politics and Health Policy: UK Health Policy in Comparative Context*, Manchester: Manchester University Press.

Hood, C.C. (1983) *The Tools of Government*, London: Macmillan.

Hudson, J. and Lowe, S. (2004) *Understanding the Policy Process*, Bristol: The Policy Press.

Jasanoff, S. (2005) *Designs on Nature: Science and Democracy in Europe and the United States*, Princeton, NJ: Princeton University Press.

Jessop, R. (2002) *The Future of the Capitalist State*, Cambridge: Polity Press.

Kingdon, J.W. (2003) *Agendas, Alternatives and Public Policies* (2nd edn), London: Longman.

Kjaer, A.M. (2004) *Governance*, Cambridge: Polity Press.

Klein, R. (1989) *The Politics of the NHS* (2nd edn), Harlow: Longman.

Lindblom, C. (1959) 'The science of muddling through', *Public Administration Review*, vol 19, pp 79-88.

Lipsky, M. (1980) *Street-level Bureaucracy: Dilemmas of the Individual in Public Services*, New York, NY: Russell Sage Foundation.

Majone, G. (1980) 'Policies as theories', *Omega: International Journal of Management Science*, vol 8, pp 151-62.

Marmor, T., Freeman, R. and Okma, K. (2005) 'Comparative perspectives and policy learning in the world of health care', *Journal of Comparative Policy Analysis*, vol 7, pp 331-48.

National Audit Office, Audit Commission and Healthcare Commission (2006) *Tackling Child Obesity: First Steps*, HC 801 Session 2005-2006, London: The Stationery Office.

Newman, J. (2001) *Modernising Governance: New Labour, Policy and Society*, London: Sage Publications.

Newman, J. (2005) 'Participative governance and the remaking of the public sphere', in J. Newman (ed) *Remaking Governance: Peoples, Politics and the Public Sphere*, Bristol: The Policy Press, pp 119-38.

Nutley, S., Walter, I. and Davies, H.W.O. (2007) *Using Evidence: How Research can Inform Public Services*, Bristol: The Policy Press.

O'Toole, L.J. Jnr (1986) 'Policy recommendations for multi-actor implementation: an assessment of the field', *Journal of Public Policy*, vol 6, H181-210.

O'Toole, L.J. Jnr (2004) 'The theory-practice issue in policy implementation research', *Public Administration*, vol 82, pp 309-29.

O'Toole, L.J. Jnr and Meier, K.J. (2003) 'Bureaucracy and uncertainty', in Barry C. Burden (ed) *Everything but Death and Taxes: Uncertainty and the Study of American Politics*, New York, NY: Cambridge University Press, pp 98-117.

Ozga, J. (2005) 'Models of policy making and policy learning', Discussion Paper 1 for Seminar on Policy Learning in 14-19 Education, Joint Seminar of Education and Youth Transition Project and Nuffield Review, University of Edinburgh.

Paton, C. (2006) *New Labour's State of Health*, Aldershot: Ashgate.

Pawson, R. and Tilley, N. (1997) *Realistic Evaluation*, London: Sage Publications.

Petticrew, M., Whitehead, M., Macintyre, S., Graham, H. and Egan, M. (2003) 'Evidence for public health policy on inequalities: 1: The reality according to policy makers', *Journal of Epidemiology and Community Health*, vol 58, pp 811-16.

PIU (Performance and Innovation Unit) (2001) *Better Policy Delivery and Design: A Discussion Paper*, London: PIU.

Pressman, J. and Wildavsky, A. (1984) *Implementation: How Great Expectations in Washington are dashed in Oakland* (3rd edn), Berkeley, CA: University of California Press.

Rein, M. (1976) *Social Science and Public Policy*, Harmondsworth: Penguin.

Rhodes, R.A.W. (1997) *Understanding Governance: Policy Networks, Governance and Accountability*, Buckingham: Open University Press.

Rittel, H., and Webber, M. (1973) 'Dilemmas in a general theory of planning', *Policy Sciences*, vol 4, pp 155-69.

Sanderson, I. (2002) 'Evaluation, policy learning and evidence-based policy making', *Public Administration*, vol 80, pp 1-22.

Saunders, P. (1979) *Urban Politics: A Sociological Interpretation*, Harmondsworth: Penguin.

Schofield, J. (2004) 'A model of learned implementation', *Public Administration*, vol 82, pp 283-308.

Schon, D.A. (1979) 'Generative metaphor: a perspective on problem-setting in social policy', in A. Ortony (ed) *Metaphor and Thought*, Cambridge: Cambridge University Press, pp 254-83.

Simon, H.A. (1982) 'From substantive to procedural rationality', in A. McGrew and M.J. Wilson (eds) *Decision Making: Approaches and Analysis*, Manchester: Manchester University Press, pp 87-96.

Sims, D. (1999) 'Organizational learning as the development of stories: canons, apochrypha and pious myths', in M. Easterby-Smith, J. Burgoyne and L. Araujo (eds) *Organizational Learning and the Learning Organization: Developments in Theory and Practice*, London: Sage Publications, pp 44-58.

Skelcher, C. (2005) 'Jurisdictional integrity, polycentrism and the design of democratic governance', *Governance*, vol 18, no 1, pp 89-110.

Sterling, R. (2005) 'Promoting democratic governance through partnerships', in J. Newman (ed) *Remaking Governance: Peoples, Politics and the Public Sphere*, Bristol: The Policy Press, pp 139-57.

Stoker, G. (1998) 'Governance as theory: 5 propositions', *International Social Science Journal*, vol 155, pp 17-28.

Thompson, J.D. (2003) *Organizations in Action: Social Science Bases of Administrative Theory*, Transaction Publishers: London.

The Times (2006) 'Child obesity grows as experts dither', 28 February.

Weiss, C.H. (1991) 'Policy research: data, ideas, or arguments?', in P. Wagner, B. Wittrock and H. Wollmann (eds) *Social Sciences and Modern States: National Experiences and Theoretical Crossroads*, Cambridge: Cambridge University Press, pp 307-32.

Weiss, C.H. (1995) 'There's nothing so useful as good theory: exploring theory-based evaluation for comprehensive community initiatives for children and families', in J.P. Connell, A.C. Kubisch, L.B. Schorr and C.H. Weiss (eds) *New Approaches to Evaluating I. Volume 1: Concepts, Methods and Contexts*, Washington, DC: Aspen Institute.

Welsh Assembly Government (2006) *Beyond Boundaries: Citizen-Centred Services for Wales. Review of Local Service Delivery: Report to the Welsh Assembly Government (Chair: Sir Jeremy Beecham)*, Cardiff: Welsh Assembly Government.

THREE

Policy innovation to tackle health inequalities

Alison Porter, Chris Roberts and Angela Clements

Introduction

The first chapter of this book reviewed the large body of evidence that we have linking inequalities in health to social structure: a link that can be most crudely summarised by saying that poor people and people living in poor places tend to die younger and live unhealthier lives than richer populations in wealthier places. The health gradient across the social classes has remained over the past hundred years or so in Britain, despite overall improvements in both health and prosperity. We know a great deal about the associations between ill health and various factors: where you live, your wealth, your position in the social hierarchy, and the lingering effects that your position in the social hierarchy in childhood can have on your health in later life (Davey Smith and Gordon, 2000). Dahlgren and Whitehead's (1991) work on the underlying determinants of health and ill health has shown how individuals, communities and society as a whole form a nested and interacting 'rainbow' of influences. We have evidence of the way in which health is unequally distributed across income gradients and across geographical areas, in the form of epidemiology and in the form of personal testimony.

While there is general consensus that the social determinants of ill health can pile on top of one another to affect our bodies in complex and accumulative ways, there is less agreement about the mechanisms by which this happens and why particular people may be affected in particular ways. The majority of work on health inequalities in the UK has explored the causal link between absolute material deprivation and health inequalities; within this strand of research, an increasing body of work is exploring the resilience of certain deprived populations, and questioning how straightforward that causal link actually is (Mitchell and Backett-Milburn, 2006). A second school of thought, following the thinking of Richard Wilkinson (Wilkinson 1996, 2005; Stewart-

Brown, 2000) emphasises the role played by relative deprivation, and argues that social and economic inequality within a state drags down the health of all, compared with those countries that are more equal.

Chapter Two argued that the relationship between a problem, a policy designed to address it and the implementation of that policy is a messy and complex one, and a subject worthy of study in its own right. This is particularly true of 'wicked problems' – intractable, multifaceted and sometimes ill-defined problems, of which health inequalities provide one important example.

Politicians, at least since the advent of New Labour government in 1997, have acknowledged that health inequalities are a problem, and have introduced various policy innovations to try to address them. This chapter provides a context for the Sustainable Health Action Research Programme (SHARP) by examining some of the policy innovations that have been put into place in the UK over the past 10 years to tackle health inequalities. It draws attention to both the complex and sometimes ad hoc processes that go on in developing and implementing policy, and to the difficulties of making choices about how to tackle such a multifaceted problem. It questions whether the policy innovations that have been introduced are necessarily the most appropriate or the most likely to be effective, and considers some of the choices that have been made in designing those interventions, in terms of underlying theory of change, breadth or narrowness of focus, and means of delivery.

The chapter goes on to describe the evolution of the SHARP initiative in Wales, highlighting the ways in which it differs from previous policy initiatives, with particular attention to characteristics that can be related to the unique structure of devolved government in Wales. It explores the origins and rationale for SHARP as a contribution to policy implementation and development. It discusses decisions about the shape of the programme, senior support and the expectations there were at the start of the programme for the kind of policy learning that would emerge. The chapter then concludes by introducing the seven projects that emerged from the selection process to be funded under SHARP.

Initiatives to tackle health inequalities
Making choices

We know that the links between health and its determinants are complex, and policy makers charged with devising interventions to reduce health inequalities have to make choices about the point at which they try to intervene. According to Diderichsen (1998), they may choose to influence the social pathways to health inequalities at any one or more of four points:

- the social position individuals occupy in society – for example, policies that impact on how long people stay in education, and thus their prospects later in life;
- exposure to health hazards faced by people in different social positions – for example, policies to improve the quality of housing;
- the effect of being exposed to a hazardous factor – for example, policies to soften or reinforce the effects of being poor;
- the impact of being ill – for example, policies affecting the equity of healthcare services.

The choice of where to intervene may be influenced by a more fundamental question, though one that is rarely articulated explicitly in research or policy literature, and that is about what underlying theories policy makers have about the mechanisms by which health inequalities can be reduced. As Carlisle (2001) has pointed out, these will in turn depend on essentially political beliefs about the determinants of health inequalities. To illustrate this, she drew on Levitas' (1998, 1999) witty model of discourses around social exclusion: RED identifies social exclusion with poverty and deprivation, MUD with a 'moral underclass' and SID with lack of social integration, specifically, with lack of paid work. Policy makers rooted in the RED discourse will attempt to tackle health inequalities by redistributing resources and reducing poverty. The MUD discourse implies interventions aimed at changing individual behaviour – encouraging people to stop smoking, for example, and generally to take responsibility for their own health. Where SID is the dominant discourse, interventions are aimed at reducing social isolation and low self-esteem through building community activity and social capital.

While the choices discussed above are the fundamental ones – the 'What?' and 'Why?' questions – there is a whole series of other choices that get made when interventions to reduce health inequalities are designed. Some of the most important of these relating to the way in which initiatives are designed, planned and managed are presented in the table below. They are all interrelated, and in turn relate to the choices made about point of intervention and underlying theories about why health inequalities exist.

Each of these choices about interventions to reduce health inequalities may be made as a matter of political expediency (Hunter, 2003).

Table 3.1: Choices in the design, planning and management of initiatives to reduce health inequalities

Focus	Does the initiative focus on health issues or on broader social/economic change? Who sets the agenda (in terms of targets and in terms of what happens)? What difference does the difference in focus make to practice?
Means of delivery and funding	Is it a framework/strategy/funding stream/self-contained project/initiative within existing service delivery? What is the role of partnership in planning and implementing the initiative?
Geography and scale	Is the initiative area-based? If so, how is the area selected and defined? What measures of health inequality (if any) are used to select the area? What impact does the choice of area have on the outcome? What learning is potentially transferable to other places, and what aspects might be unique?
Duration and sustainability	Is the project time-limited or open-ended? Is the initiative intrinsically sustainable, or will it depend on continued external support to survive? How can initiatives be sustained in the long term?
Flexibility	To what extent is the initiative working towards pre-defined targets and clear intended outcomes? How much flexibility is there to refine and change the activity and the purpose? What role do service users/citizens have in shaping the initiative?

Choices may also be influenced by pragmatic considerations (what may or may not be achievable within a short timescale, for example) or what is within the scope of a policy maker to influence (the UK national government, for example, has a different arena of influence from the Welsh Assembly Government, while the scope for action by local authorities is different again).

The next five sections of this chapter consider some of the key themes to have emerged in recent work aimed at reducing health inequalities, each reflecting what Chapter Two referred to as 'theories of change'. These themes create a bridge that transfers research findings and, indeed, policy understandings of health inequalities into objects and lines of practical action: an emphasis on individual behaviour change, a tendency to intervene 'downstream', an emphasis on area-based initiatives, the use of targets to drive interventions, and a somewhat detached relationship between the making and implementation of policy and research that aims to evaluate policy interventions. The themes are illustrated by some examples of recent interventions from Wales and other parts of the UK.

Changing individual behaviour

Whitehead (1995) reviewed the range of policy initiatives to tackle health inequalities that had been undertaken within the UK and internationally up to the early 1990s. She identified four main policy levels at which responses were designed to take effect, each one corresponding to one of the four layers of the 'rainbow' model of the determinants of health (Dahlgren and Whitehead, 1991). These layers radiate out from the individual, through communities and the environment, to the outer layer made up of macro-level influences such as the tax and welfare systems. The first two levels of policy tend to focus on disadvantaged groups or areas, while levels three and four tend to be broader. Whitehead (1995) identified an overwhelming concentration of policy at level one, but suggested that such policies to strengthen individuals need to be introduced with sensitivity to the circumstances in which people live, and to link to policies at other levels, and that:

> Some efforts also require a health warning: although they purport to empower individuals or communities, they risk being patronising and victim-blaming if not undertaken with skill and sensitivity. (Whitehead, 1995, p 51)

Despite an initial flurry of interest in structural influences on health inequalities in the early years of New Labour, the emphasis on individual behaviour change in policy at UK government level has remained, and is probably best summed up in the title of the Department of Health's White Paper, *Choosing Health* (DH, 2004). Kelly's (2004) review of public health interventions that have been shown to be effective in tackling health inequalities leans heavily towards the individual, from healthcare professionals advising people to cut down on drinking to media campaigns to increase the rate of breastfeeding. While the Welsh Assembly Government has gone further than the UK government in declaring a commitment to addressing the underlying determinants of health inequalities, much of its action has still been directed towards interventions aimed at individuals and behaviour. Health Challenge Wales was launched in 2004 as a high-profile campaign aimed at creating a climate of healthy behaviours (through exercise, good diet and caution in relation to sex, drugs and drink). Although the Assembly's promotion for the scheme emphasised the role to be taken by statutory bodies, employers and the media in making it easy for people to make healthy choices, the prime responsibility appeared to rest very clearly with the individual, with members of the public being invited to:

> ... take on the challenge to improve their health and that of their families by taking the information, advice and support available to help them to reduce their risk of future ill-health. Make their views known on what more can be done to prevent ill-health from happening in the first place – locally and nationally. (Health Challenge Wales, 2004)

This emphasis on health determinants at an individual level has drawn criticism from researchers in the field. Stewart-Brown (2000), for example, finds it remarkable that there are so many 'interventions to help poor people avoid sickness' (p 235), but not more attending to the causes of income inequality, suggesting that this subject appears to be taboo – presumably because income inequality is an expensive and politically tricky problem to address. It has also been argued that it is the fashion for evidence-based policy that has led to an inappropriate emphasis on changing individuals' behaviour, simply because such interventions are easier to measure (Frankel and Davey Smith, 1997; Davey Smith and Gordon, 2000).

The Chief Medical Officer's (CMO) emphasis on behavioural change in all aspects of life from diet to sunburn, in his *Ten Tips for Better Health* (DH, 1999), has been effectively mocked by the University of Bristol's Townsend Centre for International Poverty Research, source of much academic literature on health inequalities. The CMO's number one tip, for example, 'Don't smoke. If you can, stop. If you can't, cut down' becomes, in the Townsend (website) version, 'Don't be poor. If you are poor, try not to be poor for too long'.

Stepping in downstream

An implication of the emphasis on downstream initiatives is that the focus of action will be at local level, with 'an implicit assumption that health inequalities can be reduced without changing overall levels of inequalities' (Asthana and Halliday, 2006, p 98). Interventions aimed at modifying behaviour are far removed from the 'upstream' issues of deprivation. There is another sense, too, in which the focus of many interventions aimed at tackling health inequalities has been 'downstream', and that is that they tend to be delivered through health service providers. To be affected by these initiatives, people need to already have become patients; they need to be identified as already having poor health. The Welsh Assembly Government's Inequalities in Health Fund, for example, launched in 2001, has put £14 million into tackling coronary heart disease through 67 projects across Wales, with a strong emphasis on the promotion of personal responsibility for health (Welsh Assembly Government, 2002). Typical activities within the projects include cookery lessons from the Women's Institute (Carmarthenshire Community Heart Disease Prevention Programme) and exercise on prescription (Caerphilly, Blaenau Gwent and elsewhere). A smaller strand within the fund's work has been concerned with restructuring primary care teams to improve screening. The majority of the work of the health fund has been within health-providing organisations; although the fund was open to applications from any local government or voluntary sector organisation, as well as to NHS organisations, 94% of the projects have been led from within the NHS, mostly by local health boards. Similarly, the Healthy Communities Collaborative Programme, led by the NHS National Primary Care Development Team, has branched out into a partnership approach to tackling health inequalities from its initial brief of improving the working practice of GPs. These small-scale collaborations, established in three areas of England, have focused on two pre-determined themes – that of improving access to a healthy diet in deprived communities, and the slightly less familiar theme, in health inequalities work, or reducing falls among older people. There is a large element of peer education in both themes, for example through a buddying scheme, where people who had recovered from a fall gave one-to-one support to other older fallers to increase their confidence.

Area-based initiatives

The third overall trend in action to address health inequalities in recent years has been an emphasis on area-based initiatives (Davey Smith and Gordon, 2000). Most significant among these for health inequalities in England have been Health Action Zones (HAZs), first established in 1998 as 26 area-limited, time-limited projects. All HAZs were expected to tackle the root causes of ill health, as well as promoting community cohesion, creating opportunities for healthy lifestyles, and improving access to health services (Benzeval and Meth, 2002). Outcomes targeted for improvement by the HAZs were not necessarily specifically health outcomes – they were also to do with income, employment, social networks and so on. HAZ activities were largely characterised by partnership building and the setting of targets (Davey Smith and Gordon, 2000), rather than new, tangible service provision. One of the more lasting achievements of HAZs, it has been suggested (Armitage and Povall, 2003), will be those new linkages between communities, policy makers and professionals.

HAZs are just one member of a family of 'zone' initiatives promoted by the New Labour government, but not the only one to have some relevance to health. More recently, Local Strategic Partnerships were identified by government as a mechanism for achieving coordination in service delivery in England, with the aim of addressing a range of inequalities (Hamer and Easton, 2002). Also fitting into a declared programme of addressing the determinants of health and health inequalities were Employment Action Zones, Education Action Zones, and, particularly, Sure Start – local programmes aimed at improving the health and social development of young children in deprived areas throughout the UK. In Wales, the Communities First programme, launched in 2001, has brought regeneration funding to 132 deprived areas, through a somewhat 'top-down' approach to working with communities (Welsh Assembly Government, 2006a).

Area-based initiatives are attractive to policy makers because they provide a mechanism for limiting the scale and scope of the intervention, and bring new potential for intensive partnerships between service providers with a common interest in an area. But the example of HAZs has suggested that the use of 'area' as a targeting mechanism for interventions can be quite crude. Pockets of relative affluence and deprivation can be bundled together, and areas defined according the pre-existing service boundaries may be so large that the effectiveness of the intervention is diluted. For this and other reasons, Davey Smith and Gordon have suggested (2000, p 152) that 'area-based anti-poverty policies have a long history of only limited success or even outright failure'.

Using targets

A central plank in government policy in relation to health inequalities at both UK and Welsh Assembly Government level has been the setting of targets. These are ostensibly to be used as a (somewhat crude) measure of success, but can also play a part in defining and shaping initiatives and setting priorities for action. In 2001, the Department of Health announced two headline national targets for 2010:

• reducing inequalities in infant mortality across social groups; and
• reducing inequalities in life expectancy across social areas.

By doing so, it made a commitment to addressing *inequalities* in health rather than simply addressing poor health. These headline targets were supplemented in 2003 by a list of 12 'National Headline Indicators' on health inequalities, set out by the Department of Health in its *Tackling Health Inequalities: A Programme for Action* (DH, 2003). What is remarkable about these is that none of them is actually an indicator of ill health. One is concerned with mortality, and one with road accident casualties. The rest are concerned, more or less explicitly, with factors that are associated with health inequalities, such as 'five a day' consumption of fruit and vegetables and smoking, but are not in themselves aspects of health or illness.

Targets for change are not 'givens', but are selected. Inequalities can be measured in more than one way: making a comparison between those with the poorest health and the average may reveal very different trends from a comparison between those with the poorest health and those with the best health. The overall emphasis on inequality across social classes, with geographical inequality sometimes used as a surrogate with more emotional impact, has gone unexamined. The Black Report (DHSS, 1980) suggested that health inequalities between men and women were as great as those between men in Social Class I and Social Class V. Yet health inequalities between the genders seem to be accepted as 'normal' or inevitable, and have not been the subject of the setting of targets or associated policy interventions.

Learning from interventions

Interventions aimed at reducing health inequalities are notoriously unlikely to be effectively evaluated (Whitehead et al, 2000), in part simply because of the complexities involved and the distance between most real-life public health situations and the randomised control trial model that has favour with most health policy makers. Policy may not necessarily develop from empirical evidence, even when the political interest is there. Evidence is not always delivered at the time it is needed, and this will limit its relevance and effectiveness (Hunter, 2003).

Evidence of the effectiveness of interventions to reduce health inequalities may be hard to find and hard to handle, because of the complexities of the real-world situations in which the interventions take place (Davey Smith et al, 2001; Kelly 2004). Area-based interventions from recent years provide illustration of the difficulties of producing evidence that can feed into the development of policy with wider application. In England, the Department of Health, in partnership with the Local Government Association, has put effort into a 'pathfinder' model of learning through the Healthier Communities Shared Priority Project, aiming to provide transferable knowledge to help to narrow health inequalities. Yet so much of what happened was specific to the 12 pathfinder authorities and the structures within them that the scope for learning was limited (HDA, 2005).

Learning from interventions can also be inhibited when initiatives have to change with rapidly changing circumstances, by revising their plans and activities in response to external factors – what Bauld and Judge (2002) called, in relation to HAZs, a 'turbulent institutional and policy environment'. An extensive programme of evaluation was structured around the HAZ programme, made up of an external evaluation by a consortium of universities and, in most areas, internal evaluation by the HAZs themselves (Benzeval and Meth, 2002). Yet the majority of the HAZs, planned to last for seven years, petered out before their time was up, overtaken by changes going on around them; evaluation did not seem to influence the verdict on HAZs. By contrast, in some cases funding may be sustained for programmes where the evidence for effectiveness is equivocal, as in the case of the Sure Start local programmes (Belsky et al, 2006).

Development of the SHARP programme in Wales

The policy context in Wales

An emphasis on the underlying determinants of health and of health inequalities was a significant strand in the Welsh Assembly Government's policy in the early years of the new millennium. *Improving Health in Wales: A Plan for the NHS with its Partners* (WAG, 2001), for example, opened with a Foreword from the then Minister for Health and Social Services, Jane Hutt, which acknowledged the role of economic and social inequality in creating health inequalities:

> The experience of poverty for some of our citizens often lies at the root of ill health, unhealthy lifestyles, and contributes to a sense of hopelessness. I am determined to tackle these problems and to make progress in closing the gap between Wales and the best in Europe in relation to life expectancy, death rates from the major illnesses, and long-term illnesses. As the Plan emphasises, the social and economic determinants of ill health have often been seen as outside of the concerns of the NHS. However, the NHS in Wales will play a major role with its partners in addressing them. (WAG, 2001, p 7)

The Welsh Office's (1998) health promotion strategy, *Better Health – Better Wales* embraced the same principle of working not just towards improvements in people's health, but also towards reductions in inequalities in health. This was strongly influenced by the findings of the Wanless Report (Wanless, 2002) and its Welsh counterpart (Welsh Assembly Government, 2003), which suggested that the health of the population needed to be maintained in order to avoid a future crisis in health and social care services. At the same time, Local Health Alliances and Local Health, Social and Wellbeing Plans were two of the mechanisms introduced in Wales to encourage better partnership working between statutory providers on needs assessment, planning and service delivery. This Welsh policy context focusing on health inequalities, combined with the enthusiasm of a new Assembly keen to make its mark and an administration with a field-committed Health Promotion Division, was the fertile ground on which the SHARP initiative grew.

The aim of SHARP

It was the *Better Health – Better Wales* (Welsh Office, 1998) strategy that first highlighted the idea of a SHARP programme, later made formal in the Welsh Assembly Government's programme of action to implement the strategy (Welsh Assembly Government, 2001). The SHARP initiative was designed to show the most effective ways of breaking the cycle of poor health in Wales. The overall aim of SHARP was to establish a programme of action research to support and strengthen evidence on the effectiveness of interventions in health determinants. Within this context, the design of the SHARP programme was focused on communities with the highest incidence of ill health and premature death, social exclusion and poor life chances. In addition, the unique factor of SHARP and something that set it apart from many other community-based initiatives to improve health, such as Healthy Living Centres and Sure Start, was that it was primarily research-driven.

The centrality of the concept of action research was made explicit in the title – Sustainable Health Action Research Programme. The 'health' in the title provided the raison d'être, along with the funding, but was meant to be interpreted openly and flexibly in the implementation. The use of the word 'sustainable' was also significant: the policy makers who designed the programme were wary of introducing another set of short-term projects that would come and go without having a lasting impact.

Linking research to action in SHARP

Action research is marked by collaboration between interested practitioners, relevant organisations and communities in a cyclical investigation of issues as articulated by the participants. As discussed in Chapter Four, in traditional research the research process is separate from practice and does not involve the people for whom the problems exist in real life. In action research, an attempt is made to break down these barriers between researcher and researched by linking research directly with practice. The SHARP initiative built on the strengths of this action research approach, promoting sustainability, providing evidence of best practice at the community level, contributing to the policy development process and involving a principle of collaborative working.

The SHARP programme was made up of a series of projects across Wales, which would be based on these key requirements of partnership working and a commitment to action research. Since the action research approach was central to the development of SHARP, projects had to be made up of a multidisciplinary group of researchers and practitioners with experience of community-based working. They also had to show demonstrable partnership between the community and statutory, non-statutory, voluntary or academic sectors. Any issues that a project would address would be those that were articulated by the community or group. Projects needed to reflect the distinctive needs and circumstances of Wales; although Wales, as much as anywhere else, is heterogeneous, and the projects in the SHARP programme reflect this heterogeneity.

The SHARP programme was designed to have key research outcomes that could potentially inform policy development and future practice. These included examples of effective (and ineffective) practice in addressing health determinants and evidence of any impact of reducing health inequalities as related to the issues addressed in the participating communities. Another planned outcome was any evidence of potential for the further development of the participating communities through, for example, increased ability to complement mainstream provision, the sustainability of partnerships and increased research and other skills in the community.

Establishing and managing the SHARP programme

In designing and implementing the working format of SHARP, several options were considered, but the chosen approach was the funding of a small number of projects. It was felt that one of the key advantages of establishing a programme of projects was the synergy of bringing together a small number of communities/groups facing common issues or problems that they wanted addressed. Rather than spread the allocated money across all 22 local authorities in Wales, the Welsh Assembly Government chose instead to focus on a small number of adequately funded projects that would generate evidence.

A competitive bidding process in the spring of 2000 drew 47 applications from partnerships that were required to demonstrate collaborative working and the involvement of public, private and academic sectors in partnership with local communities. No threshold of deprivation was set for the communities for which applications were made, nor were quotas set for geographical coverage, though quite by chance the projects selected did turn out to be spread across Wales. Seven partnerships were recommended for funding by two panels of experts, one of which focused on science, and included leading academics in the field of health inequalities, and one policy panel that included people from the NHS, local government and so on.

Compared with traditional research approaches, the action research process is cyclical, sometimes spontaneous and often long term and therefore a potentially considerable administrative, monitoring and policy analysis burden. To ensure that the SHARP initiative was achieving its aims, projects were reviewed on an ongoing basis. To this end, the Welsh Assembly Government's Health Promotion Division (HPD) was responsible for the management of the SHARP programme, overseeing the day-to-day work of the projects, acting as a point of contact, monitoring budgets and dealing with any procurement or terms and conditions issues.

As part of an ongoing management and review process, regular feedback from funded projects was required. This was to monitor plans and activities against the SHARP programme's aims and objectives, with the intention of helping to identify any practice and policy lessons learnt as well as monitor and evaluate the flow of information between members of the partnership. In the interest of dissemination, projects were required to contribute to a six-monthly newsletter that was designed to update a wider audience on progress with the initiative. Project representatives were also required to attend six-monthly review meetings organised by HPD.

When the programme was designed, there was an expectation that the projects would run and be funded for up to five years. A sum of £500,000 was allocated to the SHARP initiative for each of three financial years with the first year devoted to appropriate planning and infrastructure development. Before SHARP was rolled out a donation of £10,000 was made available to help local authorities and voluntary organisations prepare for the bids and develop the infrastructure for effective implementation of the initiative. There was no specific expectation that projects would secure match funding from other sources, though there was always an intention that they would find some means to become sustainable in the long term.

With the advent of phase two, a further three years' funding of some £1.7 million was made available for 2002/03-2004/05. The seven existing projects were asked to submit proposals for phase two, anticipating that work over this period would build on the foundations established in the first phase of the research, with a particular focus on evaluating progress and assessing what projects have achieved over the course of their funding. This second phase was also dependent on output of the first phase of work, performance of the projects and the quality of project plans for phase two.

There followed a third and final phase of sustainability funding, to 2006, to support projects in further developing their local and national partnerships and networks. Sustainability of partnerships in action underpinned the aims of the SHARP initiative at phases one and two and this one-year sustainability funding was meant to ensure that key elements of partnership collaboration were sustained once core funding ended.

Outputs from the SHARP programme

An overarching evaluation of the SHARP initiative was commissioned from the Centre for Health Planning and Management at Keele University to evaluate how successfully the SHARP initiative delivered its aim and key objectives in the short, medium and, potentially, long term. The evaluation was designed to contribute to the evidence base on the effectiveness of an action research approach in tackling social determinants of health at community level and to assess the extent to which learning from the initiative was transferable to other contexts. The evaluation additionally explored how economic evaluation could be incorporated into the process.

Several other outputs, managed by the HPD team, also developed from the programme. An evaluation of the SHARP application process was undertaken to gather as much feedback on the bidding process as possible. The evaluation revealed a demand for up-to-date information on the potential for the action research approach, with particular reference to community-based health initiatives, so HPD commissioned a review of action research literature and the development of an action research resource pack. The action research literature review was published in 2003 (Whitelaw et al, 2003) and the action research resource pack published and disseminated in 2007 (Balogh et al, 2007). The resource pack is a practical guide for use by researchers, practitioners and communities across Wales on how to undertake high-quality action research, drawing on the experiences of SHARP-funded work. Both documents were in support of SHARP and aim to contribute to the development of research capacity in Wales. Finally, in order to raise awareness of the SHARP programme and its outcomes more widely, the Welsh Assembly Government commissioned a DVD featuring footage from all seven projects (Welsh Assembly Government, 2006b).

The seven SHARP projects

Holway House

The Holway is a small housing estate, predominantly in council ownership, of approximately 360 households on the outskirts of a town in Flintshire in north-east Wales. The original funding bid identified Holway as an area experiencing a range of disadvantages: high unemployment and low income, poor-quality housing, inadequate access to services and scant local participation in community activities. The bid built on preparatory community development work already undertaken by the council's Social Inclusion Unit, and the unit was the lead partner in applying for SHARP funding and acted as 'banker' for the funds once they were received.

The Holway House project converted an existing council house to a community house, which became the base for sustained community and regeneration work on the estate. SHARP funds also went towards employing a project worker, and to providing a 'partnership pot' of £12,000 a year to enable community residents to ask for and participate in activities that would otherwise be financially impossible for them. A partnership was set up to meet every six weeks to manage the project, and was made up of three key participating groups: local residents, two academic researchers, and a range of public and voluntary sector service providers. The Holway project was different from most of the SHARP programme in that there was no separate level of research or project management: all discussions and decisions took place at the partnership meetings, held in the house itself.

The activities promoted or funded by the partnership reflected the priorities of the community: seeking housing repairs and maintenance for the social housing on the estate, creating a better physical environment for the whole community, creating leisure and learning opportunities for children and adults, and trying to reduce crime and improve community safety. Grants from the 'partnership pot' went both to community groups and to individuals, to pay, for example, for driving lessons. Individuals were expected, in return, to make some contribution to one of the project's many volunteering activities, which included running a toy library and an exercise class.

In the Holway House project, the issue of 'health' was clearly located within the context of the broader social disadvantage experienced by many residents. The project placed an emphasis on building self-esteem, both as an end in itself and as a necessary forerunner of building community capacity and social capital.

Pembrokeshire: evaluating the Healthy Living Approach

The Pembrokeshire SHARP project worked with three distinct communities in west Wales: Monkton (just outside Pembroke), Hubberston and Hakin (on the outskirts of Milford Haven) and Llanychaer (a bilingual rural community near Fishguard). Pembrokeshire is traditionally a rural county, which now has considerable inward population movement. The project was concerned with developing and testing the 'Healthy Living Approach', a process of community-led needs assessment, action planning and plan implementation with a focus on health. It was led by Pembrokeshire County Council, working in partnership with health providers, academics, voluntary sector representatives and two existing community forums, one from Hubberston and Hakin and one from Monkton.

These two community forums, along with a third one developed in Llanychaer, provided the focus for the community needs assessment work undertaken by the project. Two project workers employed by the county council each combined the roles of action researcher and project coordinator. They recruited teams of local people to be trained up as community researchers, interviewing their fellow residents about their health and what they believed were the factors that influenced it. Research findings then fed in to the production of action plans by the forums, to be shared with local service providers. Like Holway, the Pembrokeshire project had a £12,000 'community chest', for community forums to access.

'Barefoot' Health Workers

The 'Barefoot' Health Workers project sought to engage some of the minority ethnic communities living in the Cardiff Bay neighbourhoods of Butetown and Grangetown in identifying, prioritising and acting on their perceived health-related needs. The project was the only one in the SHARP programme to be led by an NHS organisation, in the early stages by Cardiff's Local Health Group, and following health service restructuring in 2003, by the National Public Health Service of Wales.

Three workers, one from each of the Somali, Yemeni and Bangladeshi communities, were recruited and trained as community researchers, under the steer of a project manager. The community researchers' role was to become directly involved in researching local health needs, identifying culturally and socially appropriate ways of addressing those needs, and facilitating community involvement in developing and delivering appropriate activities.

The consultation underpinning the original bid identified five 'broad areas of need': physical activity, mental health, food and nutrition, access to health-related services and citizenship. Each of these was refined into specific themes for action. As the project developed, however, the emphasis shifted from a focus on promoting behaviour change at individual level to work directed more subtly and sensitively at the underlying determinants of health inequalities. Some of the most high-profile aspects of the project have been concerned with promoting physical activity, through, for example, women-only swimming classes, but their achievements have been wider, concerned also with building social cohesion and individual self-confidence.

Triangle

The Triangle project took its name from its work with three sites in post-industrial south Wales: the Riverside district of Cardiff, three adjacent estates in Merthyr Tydfil (the old and new Gurnos, and Galon Uchaf) and the small former coal-mining community of Ystradgynlais in Powys. The Triangle project was designed jointly by researchers at Cardiff University (the lead organisation for the bid), an independent consultancy with an interest in sustainable community regeneration and colleagues from the public health department of what was at the time Bro Taf Health Authority. They recruited four people to work on the project: a university-based researcher from south Wales who had community research experience and worked with the consultant to coordinate the project; and three researchers from the project localities who were recruited because of their local knowledge.

The original intention was to work at two levels: directly with local communities to identify key needs and concerns; and with Local Health Alliances (LHAs), newly formed multisectoral agencies with a remit to protect and improve health in their communities. However, over time, the project's role moved away from a formal relationship with LHAs, towards a more direct cycle of action and research facilitated by the three community-based action researchers, working under the project research coordinator. The Triangle project was about both gathering hitherto unavailable evidence about the character of need and potential in communities, and supporting direct response to that evidence. The Cardiff-based researcher in south Riverside also came to work closely with the researchers from the Barefoot project.

HYPP: Health of Young People in Powys

The HYPP project aimed to evaluate and facilitate effective community involvement in meeting the health needs of young people in the large rural county of Powys. It was based on the understanding that young people in rural areas have difficulties in accessing appropriate services (and so have unmet or poorly met health needs) and in achieving personal and social development. HYPP differed from most other SHARP projects in that it worked with four existing projects, rather than initiating new cycles of action and research. These four projects were:

- OASIS, a peer support health information project in Llandrindod Wells High School, later rolled out to Llanfair Caereinion High School;
- Radical, a multi-agency mobile information and advice van targeting young people;
- New Deal, a national policy initiative working with jobless young people, which included an element of advice and information; and
- the Llanwrtyd Wells Healthy Community project, which became involved in activities such as the setting-up of an alternative youth club and a youth council.

Each of these four projects had already had some involvement from young people in their development, or had identified a need to improve their structures for such involvement. During phase one of the SHARP programme, each of the four projects received £5,000 to support community development activities, which HYPP had a role in facilitating and evaluating.

HYPP was managed as a partnership between researchers at the University of Wales at Aberystwyth and the Institute of Rural Health, and local health promotion professionals. From the start, an action researcher employed by the university worked closely with a community facilitator employed by the health promotion service, and during phase two with a community worker.

Right 2 Respect

Right 2 Respect (R2R) was a project for girls and young women in Wrexham county borough. It was both an evaluation of existing provision for young people and a new project in its own right, setting up six groups across the Wrexham area that combined action research and youth work. The origins of R2R lay in the Education and Leisure Directorate of Wrexham County Borough Council, and over its life it became embedded in and 'owned' by the council's Youth and Community Services department. It provides a marked contrast with Holway and Pembrokeshire, both of which were ostensibly led by their local council but operated in seeming isolation.

The project targeted girls and young women in the age group 11-25, and aimed to bring about change at three levels: by developing skills and social networks among individuals, by improving services through more effective user involvement and evaluation, and by developing a model of work that could inform policy.

The project was run day to day by a young female project coordinator with a background in youth and community work, and delivered by a team of project workers. Academic support was provided by the University of Wales, Bangor. Over phase two of the SHARP programme, the team gradually withdrew from basic delivery of young women's sessions in youth clubs and centres across the area to focus more on working in partnership with the youth service's training team to 'spread the R2R ethos' to both female and male youth workers across the area.

BeWEHL

The Bettws Women's Education, Health and Lifestyle project (BeWEHL) was based on a disadvantaged housing estate on the edge of Newport, and worked exclusively with women. It was set up as a partnership between the University of Wales, Newport and the Workers' Educational Association (WEA). The project aimed to evaluate what impact adult education had on the wellbeing of women who took part in it.

Women taking part in the project had a dual role: they learned research skills that enabled them to take part in research projects on the estate, and they were themselves part of the action research process, in that the personal impact of the project on their lives was one of the potential outcomes of the project. Involvement was staged, with participants starting off by spending a year in 'MAD' – the Making A Difference group. From here they could, if they wished, progress to spending a year as BeWEHL co-researchers, attending project sessions at the university, before finally becoming 'FEDs' – further education students. As it developed, the project spread beyond the community of Bettws and, while it kept its acronym, changed its full name to 'Bettering Women's Education, Health and Lifestyles'.

Conclusion

Across Wales and the UK as a whole, the picture of policy initiatives addressing health inequalities is a busy one. Action is being taken in terms of target setting, establishment of partnerships and funding, and on-the-ground activity, but it tends to be area-based rather than implemented evenly across the country. Even within areas of a reasonable size – such as the HAZs – particular projects may be limited to particular neighbourhoods. Rather than one overall programme of work, there is a large number of 'little hits'. On average, projects have tended to be time-limited and target-driven. There is a mixed story about evaluation: it has been carried out in some, but not all, cases, and the relationship between evaluation and policy continuation or development is not always clear. It is not possible to look at the case studies of interventions to tackle health inequalities and say which is the most effective.

None of the initiatives described appears to have resolved the tension between the 'top-down' imposition of policy and targets, and the need to find 'bottom-up' solutions that are appropriate to the communities involved. For all the government's emphasis on the need for community participation and involvement, health inequalities work appears to be led much more strongly by external agents than by communities. Projects may intersect, in terms of area or target group, but not necessarily interact, and the amount of time and effort that goes – repeatedly – into building partnerships, and succeeding minimally or failing completely can be quite depressing. Moreover, for the agencies themselves, under all kinds of other pressures, it is also the case that failing to achieve improvements on one or other measure of health inequalities is not necessarily a crucial issue: there are other things that will make the difference in terms of keeping or losing your job.

SHARP has fitted in with the mainstream of work to tackle health inequalities in some respects, in particular, by having an area-based focus, and by promoting partnership working. In other respects, though, it does swim against the tide: it is not structured around targets, it does not start with a pre-determined model of how change will be brought about, and it has built the research and evaluation component directly into the process, rather than having it as an 'add-on'. Most strikingly, it represents a daring move by a government organisation to adopt a mode of working – action research – that is traditionally associated with challenges to authority and fundamental change.

Born of seven very different partnerships, the seven SHARP projects varied not just in the practical content of their work but also in terms of the way in which they theorised the pathways leading to health inequalities, which are also the pathways along which interventions can be made. In the next section of the book we explore the experience of the SHARP projects in more detail, looking at the success with which the projects managed genuinely and sustainably to engage local people and really make partnership across agencies work.

References

Armitage, M. and Povall, S. (2003) 'Practical issues in translating evidence into policy and practice', in A. Oliver and M. Exworthy (eds) *Health Inequalities: Evidence, Policy and Implementation*, London: Nuffield Trust.

Asthana, S. and Halliday, J. (2006) *What Works in Tackling Health Inequalities? Pathways, Policies and Practice through the Lifecourse*, Bristol: The Policy Press.

Balogh, R., Markwell, S. and Watson, J. (2007) *Action Research Resource Pack*, Cardiff: Welsh Assembly Government.

Bauld, L. and Judge, K. (eds) (2002) *Learning from Health Action Zones*, Chichester: Aeneas Press.

Belsky, J., Melhuish, E., Barnes, J., Leyland, A.H. and Romaniuk, H. (2006) 'Effects of Sure Start local programmes on children and families: early findings from a quasi-experimental, cross-sectional study', *British Medical Journal*, vol 332, pp 1476-8.

Benzeval, M. and Meth, F. (2002) 'Innovation', in L. Bauld and K. Judge (eds) *Learning from Health Action Zones*, Chichester: Aeneas Press.

Carlisle, S. (2001) 'Inequalities in health: contested explanations, shifting discourses and ambiguous policies', *Critical Public Health*, vol 11, no 3, pp 267-81.

Dahlgren, G. and Whitehead, M. (1991) *Policies and Strategies to Promote Social Equity in Health*, Stockholm: Institute for Future Studies.

Davey Smith, G. and Gordon, D. (2000) 'Poverty across the lifecourse and health', in C.Pantazis and D. Gordon (eds) *Tackling Inequalities: Where are We Now and What can be Done?* Bristol: The Policy Press.

Davey Smith, G., Ebrahim, S. and Frankel, S. (2001) 'How policy informs the evidence', *British Medical Journal*, vol 322, pp 184-5.

DH (Department of Health) (1999) *Saving Lives: Our Healthier Nation*, London: DH.

DH (2003) *Tackling Health Inequalities: A Programme for Action*, London: DH.

DH (2004) *Choosing Health: Making Healthy Choices Easier*, Cm 6374, London: DH.

DHSS (Department of Health and Social Security) (1980) *Inequalities in Health: Report of a Working Group* (the Black Report), London: DHSS.

Diderichsen, F. (1998) 'Understanding health equity in populations: some theoretical and methodological considerations', in *Promoting Research on Inequalities in Health: Proceedings from an International Expert Meeting*, Stockholm: Swedish Council for Social Research.

Frankel, S. and Davey Smith, G. (1997) 'Evidence-based medicine and treatment choices', *The Lancet*, vol 349 issue 9051, p 571.

Hamer, L. and Easton, N. (2002) *Community Strategies and Health Improvement: A Review of Policy and Practice*, London: Health Development Agency.

HDA (Health Development Agency) (2005) *The Healthier Communities Shared Priority Project: Learning from the Pathfinder Authorities*, London: HDA.

Health Challenge Wales (2004) http://new.wales.gov.uk/topics/health/improvement/hcw/?lang=en (accessed in 2004; website since updated).

Hunter, D. (2003) *Public Health Policy*, Cambridge: Polity Press.

Kelly, M. (2004) *The Evidence of the Effectiveness of Public Health Interventions – and the Implications*, HDA Briefing No 1, London: Health Development Agency.

Levitas, R. (1998) *The Inclusive Society? Social Exclusion and New Labour*, Basingstoke: Macmillan.

Levitas, R. (1999) 'Defining and measuring social exclusion: a critical overview of current proposals', *Radical Statistics*, vol 71, pp 10-27.

Mitchell, R. and Backett-Milburn, K. (2006) *Health and Resilience: What does a Resilience Approach offer Health Research and Policy?*, Research Findings 11, Edinburgh: Research Unit in Health, Behaviour and Change, University of Edinburgh.

Stewart-Brown, S. (2000) 'What causes social inequalities in health?', *Critical Public Health*, vol 10, pp 233-42.

Townsend Centre for International Poverty Research (no date) 'The Chief Medical Officer's ten tips for better health and our alternative tips', www.bristol.ac.uk/poverty/health%20inequalities.html (accessed 28 August 2007).

Townsend, P., Davidson N. and Whitehead, M. (1988) *Inequalities in Health: The Black Report and the Health Divide*, Harmondsworth: Penguin.

Wanless, D. (2002) *Securing our Future Health: Taking a Long-term View*, London: HM Treasury.

Welsh Assembly Government (2001) *Improving Health in Wales: A Plan for the NHS with its Partners*, Cardiff: Welsh Assembly Government.

Welsh Assembly Government (2002) *The Inequalities in Health Fund: An Interim Evaluation Report*, Cardiff: Welsh Assembly Government.

Welsh Assembly Government (2003) *Review of Health and Social Care in Wales – The Report of the Project Team advised by Derek Wanless*, Cardiff: Welsh Assembly Government.

Welsh Assembly Government (2006a) *Interim Evaluation of Communities First: Final Report*, Cardiff: Welsh Assembly Government.

Welsh Assembly Government (2006b) 'SHARP: working together to improve our lives', DVD Dart Film and Video, Cardiff: Welsh Assembly Government.

Welsh Office (1998) *Better Health – Better Wales*, Cm 3922, Cardiff: The Stationery Office.

Whitehead, M. (1995) 'Tackling health inequalities: a review of policy initiatives', in M. Benzeval, K. Judge and M. Whitehead (eds) *Tackling Inequalities in Health: An Agenda for Action*, London: King's Fund.

Whitehead, M., Diderichsen, F. and Burström, B. (2000) 'Researching the impact of public policy on inequalities in health', in H. Graham (ed) *Understanding Health Inequalities*, Maidenhead: Open University Press.

Whitelaw, S., Beattie, A., Balogh, R. and Watson, J. (2003) *A Review of the Nature of Action Research*, Cardiff: Welsh Assembly Government.

Wilkinson, R. (1996) *Unhealthy Societies: The Afflictions of Inequality*, London: Routledge.

Wilkinson, R. (2005) *The Impact of Inequality: How to Make Sick Societies Healthier*, London: Routledge.

FOUR

Action research partnerships: contributing to evidence *and* intelligent change

*Steve Cropper, Helen Snooks, Angela Evans, Janet Pinder
and Kevin Shales*

Introduction

The use of action research to inform and develop public policy and professional practice has a long tradition. Its roots can be found in a variety of intellectual traditions and practices. In the analysis of conflict between social groups, where the method originated (Lewin, 1948), in industry, where programmes of work on industrial democracy and quality of working life were pursued by the Tavistock Institute of Human Relations (Rapoport, 1970), and in health and social care (Winter and Munn-Giddings, 2001), where Hart and Bond (1995) published a comprehensive account, action research has become well recognised as a method for learning and change. Lewin's own work and stance on action research and on social (field) theory for change has been examined, challenged and positively reassessed (Burnes, 2004). Thriving specialist centres of teaching and practice and a growing range of publications add to debate about the character of action research and its relationship to other forms of inquiry and practice. The publication of an academic handbook dedicated to action research (Reason and Bradbury, 2001) is testimony to the extent of interest in the approach and its growing maturity.

As commentaries on the approach suggest, and as we will explain and illustrate below, action research has developed a range of forms, each emphasising different commitments within a complex and contingent practice. There is a set of basic, shared commitments: to linking inquiry and intervention to produce intelligent action for change; to iteration between action and research in a spiral or helical process; to seeking to develop understanding progressively during the course of the process; to create the conditions where action can take place and be revised; and to collaborative inquiry involving practitioners and researchers.

But there are also choices to be made and tensions that arise in the organisation, design and practice of action research and this chapter reflects on choices made and tensions experienced in the projects in the Sustainable Health Action Research Programme (SHARP).

Chapter Two argued that, while there is a great deal of evidence about the social patterning and causes of health inequalities, there is much less evidence about how practically to address inequalities, especially through local action, and what the costs and 'side effects' of policies/ actions might be. In Chapter Three, we argued that, for the originators and commissioners of SHARP, action research offered a means of drawing together the efforts of a variety of interests – researchers, policy makers and public service organisations and professionals, and members of communities – in exploring two questions:

- What might be involved in addressing the wider determinants of health at local level?
- What lessons can be drawn to help in breaking the cycle of poor health and inequalities in health in Wales?

The method is well suited to situations in which the effectiveness of means to given ends is uncertain and in particular to the bottom right-hand cell of the matrix shown in Table 2.1 (page 32), where there is uncertainty about both purpose and means.

The focus of this chapter is to draw out learning from SHARP about how it might be possible to organise and undertake action research so that there is both immediate benefit to the local community and relevant learning. Although there has been much recent attention to questions of community development, governance and partnership (Gittell and Vidal, 1998; Trevillion, 1999; Balloch and Taylor, 2001, and so on), there has been less discussion of the place of research in these processes. We take as our cue, therefore, Mayo's (1974) conclusion about the potential of community development to promote concerted and inclusive analysis of change and the questions she poses about

> the role of research from the perspective of the community worker in the field ... in assisting a community in the diagnosis of the underlying causes of its problems.... Nor is there adequate discussion of the role of research in relation to strategic planning, once this initial process of problem identification and analysis has taken place: the point at which the role of research merges with that of the community workers themselves, as a research and

development unit of the community in which they work. (Mayo, 1974, pp 243-4)

We return to these points – the character of action, its relationship to research and inquiry, and the organisation of each – throughout the discussion of SHARP's experience with local, community-based action research.

Although it has seldom taken centre stage in the way that it did in SHARP, there are some precedents for the use of action research in addressing inequalities and there are some lessons to be drawn from those experiences that will help to set SHARP in context. In the 1970s, the Home Office-sponsored programme of Community Development Programmes (CDPs), largely set in cities, sought to fuse inquiry and action to redress the effects of industrial restructuring and social change in Britain. The projects broke up, or were closed down early, as the realisation grew that these efforts at neighbourhood level to tackle fundamental processes of change, decline and exclusion were unrealistic. What could be addressed at the local level, however, were the compounding effects of local agencies, both in terms of their assumptions about communities and their problems, and their assumptions about potential interventions. In order to bring change to the delivery of services the better to meet local need, there was a shift in focus from community to local institutions and their failure. But it was recognised that this would not be 'quick work' or easy work, particularly where it required the redistribution of resources. Following on from this, the role of 'intermediary' between local agencies and communities gave way to a more politicised advocacy, identifying 'strategies for injecting our small-scale commentary into arteries of the wider debate' (Benington, 1974, p 276). This sought to contribute to what Benington later termed 'propositional' rather than 'oppositional' planning. Action research could, then, play a role in assisting

> local groups to decide what they are for, not just what they are against. It has to try to identify and develop the common interests within diverse and sometimes divided communities…. The second task is more difficult – how to link local government in to these complex grassroots communities. (Benington, 1997, pp 239-40)

A decade before the English CDPs, the US poverty programme had also sought to bring social science to bear to inform action in each of its local projects. The evaluators of this programme, Peter Marris and Martin Rein (1967), reflected on the limitations of the approach:

> After five years of effort, the reforms had not evolved any reliable solutions to the intractable problems with which they struggled. They had not discovered how in general to override the intransigent autonomy of public and private agencies, at any level of government; nor how to use the social sciences practically to formulate and evaluate policy; nor how, under the sponsorship of government, to raise the power of the poor.... The search for coherence, knowledge and a viable organization of the poor was still perplexed by inherent contradictions. (Marris and Rein, 1967, pp 222-3)

Although the scope of partnerships for social action was in many senses impressive, the contradictions Marris and Rein noted were a consequence of the different jurisdictions, interests and purposes that each of the partners brought to the task, as well as the social, economic and political conditions of 'the poor'. In the end, as Benington later concluded for the British CDP, they find that there is scope for local action and for learning that has wider impact:

> even if the ideal is ultimately unrealizable, at least in these five years community action developed a range of skills, concepts, organizations, models of action, which equipped the search with much more sophisticated means. And by this it had already stimulated a realignment of resources and ideas which powerfully influenced the variety of initiatives that now competed for priority in the exploration of reform. (Marris and Rein, 1967, p 223)

These uses of action research in promoting learning about public policy and community development/action on deprivation suggest that *both positive change and learning* can result from interventionist social science at community level. The claim has been that the most significant value ultimately lies in the wider diffusion of learning – about the experience and causes of deprivation or exclusion, the ways in which local institutional practices and the organisation of national policy collude to reinforce and sustain inequalities. Yet learning cannot occur without effective access – to the experience of life in excluded communities, where inequalities bear most evidently, and to the local institutions that have responsibility for the administration of welfare services, the promotion of democratic debate and the local response to inequalities.

This chapter sets out some aspects of the experience of action research that sought to engage directly and wholeheartedly with communities and, through partnerships with local agencies both directly and indirectly, in a process of inquiry and action. First, we reprise the character of action research, particularly participatory action research. We then consider the experience of action research in SHARP, discussing how action research was conceived variously, the balance struck and relationships forged between action and research, and the contexts of partnership in which the projects sought to engage. Finally, we make brief comment on the organisation of action research – the possibilities for division of labour across participants.

Characteristics of action research

One of the founders of the action research approach, Kurt Lewin, defined it as:

> comparative research on the conditions and effects of various forms of social action, and research leading to social action. Research that produces nothing but books will not suffice. (Lewin, 1948, pp 202-3)

Subsequent definitions have expanded on this:

> Action research can be described as a family of research methodologies which pursue action (or change) and research (or understanding) at the same time ... using a cyclic or spiral process which alternates between action and critical reflection ... continuously refining methods, data and interpretation in the light of the understanding developed in the earlier cycles. It is thus an emergent process which takes shape as understanding increases. It is an iterative process which converges towards a better understanding of what happens. In most of its forms it is also participative and qualitative. (Dick, 1999)

If definitions of the approach vary, the practice of action research also varies. Heller (1993) suggested that the variety could be reduced to two forms, 'action research' and 'research action'. Chandler and Torbert (2003), however, offer 27 different 'flavours' of action research. In their useful and influential analysis, Hart and Bond (1995) propose a spectrum of types of action research. This ranges from 'experimental' to 'empowerment' models and suggests that movement from one end of the spectrum to the other is characterised by different emphases – experimental action research gives greater prominence to research;

empowerment action research privileges 'action' as the prime outcome of the approach.

Cassell and Johnson (2006) argue that the variety of forms of action research reflects the range of different philosophical assumptions on which method and practice are built. Thus, experimental action research is based on a view of the world as knowable through the observation of facts that allow propositions about cause–effect relationships between variables to be verified or proved false. Action research is a means of testing theories that bear on social problems – theory is taken into the field and 'cause' and 'effect' become equivalent to 'means' and 'end' (see Rein (1976) for a critique of this position). Adjacent forms of action research emphasise learning from ongoing practice rather than tight, theory-oriented experiments – observations or experiences in the field suggest theories through processes of analysis or reflection, respectively. The action researcher remains the 'expert knowledge worker'.

With such differences in emphasis, it is not unexpected that action research makes use of a range of research designs, methods and techniques. There are, though, five characteristics that are found, to a greater or lesser extent, in all action research projects.

First, *action research seeks directly to link, and potentially to fuse, primary inquiry and intervention*. Research – we will also use the term 'inquiry' – can be used in a variety of ways to inform, guide and design, track, record and evaluate action. There is a fundamental tension between the pursuit of change and the generation of knowledge in action research (Rapoport, 1970; Eden and Huxham, 1996). This raises questions of purpose, design and how to understand the social and material conditions within which the possibilities for change are considered and action occurs. Though Lewin famously noted that 'there's nothing so practical as a good theory', he was also clear that general laws do not prescribe the strategy for change; they do not necessarily help to understand what conditions exist locally at a given place at a given time, and do not do the job of diagnosis, which has to be done locally.

Second, *the emergent character of action research* is therefore given prominence in certain accounts, in which early experience and results shape the subsequent direction of the inquiry process and its associated action – a so-called 'cycle' or 'spiral'. The cyclical nature of the action research process is illustrated in Figure 4.1, which is modified from Susman's (1983) original model in that his central, linking concept of 'developing a client system infrastructure' is replaced here by that of 'developing and managing relationships with multiple participants'.

Third, *understanding in action research takes shape progressively*, as the nature and significance of action are clarified and as participants and

Figure 4.1: The cyclical processes of action research

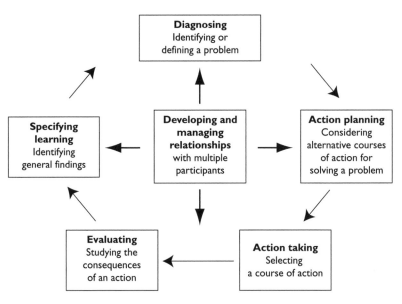

Source: adapted from Susman (1983)

stakeholders converge towards a richer, more confident account of what has been tried, achieved and learned. This is in marked contrast to conventional research projects, where research processes are tightly designed and rigorously conducted, and 'findings' emerge at the end.

This direct and immediate relationship between action and inquiry distinguishes action research from many other forms of research and from professional practices that rely, for example, on declared plans or on laws, rules and conventions to guide action. Proposals for public funding – including, for example, regeneration projects – have tended to require 'delivery plans', which set out in advance what is to be achieved and against which projects will be held to account. Research protocols, too, will often have to specify what is to be done, how many heads will be counted. But prior understanding is not always adequate to specify in advance what will be important, or what the interventions should be, and different ideas about 'what would work' to promote change for the better will probably surface. Following recent thinking in evaluation methodology, we can call such hunches, beliefs, ideas for action and hypotheses 'theories'. In using the word 'theory', we do not mean grand social science, but, rather, the way in which we make sense of our worlds – what is wrong, why we have arrived there, why it is not acceptable, and what might change things for the better.

Fourth, in action research the task is *to create the conditions in which it is possible to generate action, and where there is also time and space to observe what happens and to adjust, extend or change the nature of the action.* Sandberg (1985) and Kemmis (2001) emphasise the dialogical or discursive character of action research. The focus might start with the recognition or identification of a problem, but usually there is also a 'plausible' idea (or many) about what to do. The question might be whether it is possible to get the idea into action at all and what, practically, it means, but action research will tend also to ask whether the action delivered effects that we thought were good and useful. Action research is a chance to look hard at the theories that form and govern our practice and, where the results justify it, to give them a real sense of life precisely because they have been challenged. In sum, the purpose of action research is to create the conditions in which to explore, articulate and challenge our theories.

Finally, *action research is collaborative,* in more than one way. It extends the relationship with a community beyond the question of access to a 'site for experimentation'. Stringer's (1996) account of community-based action research emphasises the commitment to 'a non-traditional approach where the researcher and subject/participant become co-researchers through an interactive relationship of enquiry' (p 9). As the spectrum of types of action research practice shifts to participatory action research, and into research that is committed primarily to empowerment and social critique, the place of knowledge and the action researcher as observer becomes fully entwined with social practices.

Action research is also collaborative in the sense of building links between practitioner and researcher roles. Action research is thus presented as an ongoing process of negotiation between researchers and those responsible for action, rather than something that is proposed, and then taken or left. Indeed, although some action researchers do make a strong distinction between theoretical and practitioner knowledge interests and products (for example, Eden and Huxham, 1996; Huxham and Vangen, 2003), the practical orientation and the experiential knowledge of practitioners may well be given equal or even privileged status in the joint inquiry (Reason, 1994). Whyte (1991, p 7) defines this in terms of the involvement of practitioners 'in the research process from the initial design of the project, through data gathering and analysis to final conclusions and actions arising out of the research'. In this version of action research, local knowledge, professional and lay, is not only for 'consumption' by researchers, but is fundamentally a part of the construction of theories of practice – of problems and of interventions. Research, then, should be supportive of practitioner theorising and intervention. Since the claim is that action research provides a method for generating valid knowledge through action, establishing the proper status and character of that knowledge is a key task.

However, if practitioners are assumed to have an equal status in working knowledge in action research, it is also the case that researchers, as Benington's (1974) account made clear, might also find that they are taken beyond their normal responsibilities to become participants in action – as change agents, mobilising, advocating and influencing. With this sharing, if not integration, of roles, come responsibilities – social, ethical and practical (Hammersley, 1999). Accounts of action research argue, both from fundamental values and from the practical question of maintaining effective relations, that the approach should involve the creation and maintenance of social and personal interactions that are both non-exploitative and pursued in such a way as to enhance participants' social and emotional lives. Indeed, many accounts of action research emphasise the importance of collaborative or participative inquiry in which control of action and control of the design and conduct of inquiry are both intimately related and 'shared' among participants. The approach is thus thought to have the potential – perhaps absent from more traditional ('extractive') modes of research – for greater sensitivity, connection and responsiveness to local purpose and context; for realising local potential and contributing to local 'capacity'; and finally, through its impact on the organisation of local activity, for mobilising longer-term impact and promoting sustainability (Reason, 1994; Hart and Bond, 1995; Boutilier et al, 1997; Waterman et al, 2001).

A recent review of action research in healthcare (Waterman et al, 2001)) identified a number of positive aspects of the action research approach, including understanding of context, problem identification by participants, development of appropriate and feasible innovations, provision of educational opportunities, and ownership allowing rapid uptake of change. However, the authors identified negative aspects, too: disruption of existing boundaries of decision making; initiation of shifts in existing relationships; requirement for energy to maintain activities and capacities; opportunity for domination by more powerful participants; need for time to realise outcomes; creation of resistance to change; and negative feelings if change is not implemented. The identification of these social and political aspects of action research experience as negative is telling. One purpose of participative action research is to provide a legitimate, intelligent basis on which to generate change. This involves the production of evidence for change – what Lewin called 'diagnosis' – but there is also a responsibility to create the conditions in which action for change can occur. Only as planned change occurs can the action research cycle and the learning process be completed.

Action research in SHARP

Conceptions of action research across SHARP

If action research can take such a variety of forms, what, then, has been the set of principles guiding SHARP projects? And what has been the experience and value felt by participants and commissioners of using action research? The SHARP programme and its projects were ambitious in many ways – not just in their focus on learning about how inequalities might be addressed at the local level, but also in the ways in which they conceived of institutional change, and in the extent of change they believed might be possible in the three years initially available following the 'start-up period'. Universally, the conception of action research was of a collaborative process of inquiry in which members of communities, public policy and service organisations and academic researchers worked together to produce evidence about how to address health inequalities through local action. There was relatively little experience among professional and academic partners of action research and the projects' initial conceptions of this mode of inquiry were in some cases quite radically revised.

In making their proposals, the projects were asked to indicate not only how they would initiate action to address health inequalities through their partnerships, but also how they would evaluate the outcomes of their work. In responding, projects made a number of fundamental assumptions: about the way health inequalities might be manifest and seen as tractable at local level; about the nature of communities; and about the nature and relevance of action research. In this chapter, we focus on the last of these, although we also try to indicate how the design and practice of action research depends on how community, 'the problem' and scope of responsibility are understood.

Project teams worked hard to establish an interpretation of action research, at times seeking reassurance or support from academic advisers/members that 'what we're doing is right – in that it's about not being scared of things going wrong'. The Welsh Assembly Government had commissioned a review of the literature on action research and this had been circulated to projects (Whitelaw et al, 2003), together with a draft action research resource pack (Balogh et al, 2004). Despite

—

this guidance, which recognised the diversity of possible form and practice in action research, projects had to work through their own uncertainties about how action research would be conducted. These were of three types:

- the uncertainty as to what counts as action research – is it about systematic data gathering and action or a looser cycle of organising and action and personal/collective reflection on that action?;
- the uncertainty as to what is being researched/evaluated – specific activities and their outcomes, or the process of identifying priorities and mobilising for activities, or the character and value of action research more generally?;
- the uncertainty as to where and when research happens – all the time, on everything, or episodically on discrete activities, or after a build-up of action on particular issues?

SHARP's experience suggests that action research in the context of community work is likely to become closely entwined with, and difficult to separate from, community development activity. Multiple research methods are deployed to elicit community members' understandings of factors that influence health and wellbeing for good or ill, and to facilitate local involvement in action to address these. The Holway House project spelled this out in a 'how to' guide to action research, which was displayed prominently on the wall in the main community room of the project house, and is reproduced in Figure 4.2. The guide was constructed by the local community development worker and researchers.

Despite this visible reminder, action research as such was rarely discussed in Holway partnership meetings. Given the emphasis on community development by the lead partner and the funding of a post for this specific purpose, action research *as a conscious activity* tended to be conducted by the two academics involved. This does not mean that action research did not happen on Holway, but it does suggest that it took a less visible form. Projects that attempt to work in genuine (rather than tokenistic) partnership with the community are obliged to pay attention to community priorities in order to retain credibility and maintain good working relationships.

Figure 4.2: The Holway House project action research model

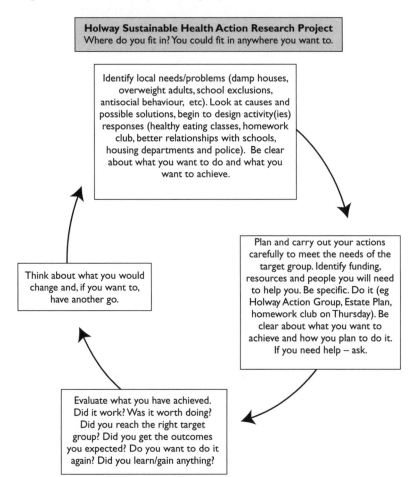

The conduct of action research: Holway

During a summer Youth Challenge, one of the Holway project researchers was trying to obtain children's views on how the estate had changed/if things had improved, over the life of the SHARP project. Although something of a captive audience (they were painting seashells to decorate bollards outside the Community Centre), they seemed to find the questions either very difficult to answer or simply irrelevant and tended to wander off when interest waned. Nor did the adult participants seem to want to reflect in any depth on activities: judgements of success or failure are made in swift and simple terms.

For people living in the Holway neighbourhood, action *research* was not the highest priority. The main exception to this occurred when a number of residents willingly joined the academic researchers to conduct a local housing condition survey, a priority issue for the community. With the researchers, they presented their findings to the housing maintenance department of the council. These were not well received: survey respondents had been blunt in their criticisms of the housing maintenance service and service providers reacted defensively at first, even to the extent of questioning whether the survey was 'truthful'. Promises were made, but have never been kept, of regular meetings with community residents and updates of maintenance and repair programmes. Changes in senior personnel within the council have also partly militated against effective action in this instance, as has the sheer scale and cost of the necessary repairs.

Striking a balance between action and research

While action research must, by definition, contain elements of both action and research, there are now absolute rules about how these are to be linked. The 'action' part of the process does not necessarily have to be integral to or contained within the project, but might be achieved through partnership. Two of the SHARP projects chose not to integrate action directly into the research process. The Pembrokeshire SHARP was originally proposed as an evaluation of a Healthy Living Centre; when that initiative did not materialise, the project sought to test a 'healthy living approach' through using action research as an evaluation tool, but with no 'focal investment' to initiate and develop change. Surveys of community health and wellbeing at the start and end of the project time frame would measure change over time and would also serve as an evidence base for local communities and policy makers to assess need, devise appropriate responses and select priorities. The project would observe rather than assert itself into the action. It would undertake evaluation of activities or interventions that were already in place or planned.

HYPP (Health of Young People in Powys) drew on a model of action research as evaluation in selecting existing service initiatives for young people in rural Powys. A school-based peer counselling and support service (OASIS project), a health bus (RADICAL) and

New Deal for Young People – a project aimed at improving chances of employment – were projects that seemed on the face of it to hold out prospects both for learning about how to respond effectively to the challenges of rural provision for young people and, because they were existing commitments made by local service organisations, for sustained provision. Difficulties in accessing appropriate services and in achieving personal and social development meant that questions of service reach and sensitivity to the experience of young people were crucial. A key issue identified was young people's relative lack of capacity to articulate needs and change this situation. HYPP also sought to build, through partnership work among the major agencies, greater responsiveness both to evidence about the needs of young people and to assessment of what works. Although HYPP's role was to provide, or to orchestrate provision of, such evidence and assessment, in two cases this involved more than research. HYPP provided resources and support to the school-based counselling service while it re-established itself, and the project helped to initiate and establish a youth council, recognised by its adult counterpart, as a means of ensuring that young people's views would be represented and heard.

By contrast, other projects took a view that a primary function would be to initiate action as a basis for their research. Their starting point was a recognition that:

> Decades of purportedly benevolent research and regeneration activities are perceived to have made little contribution to the improvement of the social and economic conditions of these communities and, some might argue, have further stigmatised them. (Triangle, 2005)

Recognising that 'initiative fatigue' is as much of a problem as 'research fatigue', when trying to engage with communities, there was an emphasis on investment in change that was designed to be sustainable. The communities with which the projects were engaged would be encouraged to articulate their needs and preferences and to take part in the development and delivery of activities, services and change with the appropriate local agencies. An insistence on participatory practice was central. In particular, projects argued that participation was essential if activities and investments were to respect and respond to the character of the community, if they were to recognise the history and experience of the previous initiatives, if they were to engage local people because they were more sensitive to communities' own forward-looking definition of their needs. There was also a sense, especially early in the projects' lives, that activities should evidently and even unconditionally be responsive to locally expressed needs. Research methods and practices could help to explore the nature, shape and history of the communities. Through research it would be possible to: gather, measure and make sense of the community's needs; to identify assets (resources and activities) that people felt were of value or could be developed, and other opportunities for change; and to assess existing policy and provision. Although there was a strong tendency for members of communities, and of agencies too, to focus on action, the SHARP projects found a variety of ways of encouraging and developing participation in the research process. In doing this, the projects also sought a longer-term outcome – change in the way agencies and partnerships related to those communities.

In Right 2 Respect (R2R), needs assessment was seen as a first stage in the process of provoking change in services provided: girls and young women, potentially at risk from processes of social exclusion, were asked to identify issues important to them. Training in interview methods would also allow this group to consult with their peers and so assess what issues were of relevance to the broader young female community. Opportunities to undertake action research training would also be offered to staff from health, local authority and voluntary agencies: it was assumed that this would encourage others to adopt the approach and spread it beyond the confines of the one project. Findings generated through this action research process would inform a conference for dissemination/future planning purposes, providing recommendations for improved service provision or specific activities. It was assumed that service providers would implement and review, with service users, such recommendations.

Triangle aimed to inform and influence the policies of newly emerging partnerships about health and wellbeing in post-industrial communities through highly engaged research, with community researchers invited to identify community priorities for action and to initiate project and wider responses. The 'Barefoot' Health Workers project, working with minority ethnic communities in Cardiff, also employed community researchers recruited from those communities to draw up an 'insider' account that would deepen an earlier needs assessment conducted by health promotion professionals.

SHARP projects tended to espouse both experimental and empowering elements of action research. Action would be established in response to expressions of need by the focus communities that had been elicited and reported by the research element of the project, which would then evaluate the extent to which the intervention made a difference. The conventional action research 'cycle' starts with 'reconnaissance', moves to 'research' and 'action', and then to 'evaluation and gathering learning' (see, for example, Hart and Bond, 1995). But action research is messier than that. Reconnaisance may suggest some immediate actions that may bypass the research phase straight to action. Research may not indicate what to do. Action may not happen, at least as intended. Both research and action would be opportunities to encourage, extend and deepen the resources within communities, including, most importantly, human and social capital. The BeWEHL project, for example, was set up to test the impact of access to adult education on health and wellbeing (an experimental aim), but its desired outcomes clearly involved enhancing self-esteem and confidence among participants (an empowering goal).

In sum, the patterns of action research in SHARP have been varied, and since projects have commonly carried a variety of forms of action and research at any time, complex action research cycles have been both long run and short run. Pembrokeshire's community surveys took some four years to complete and to translate into community-owned action plans and a basis for advocacy with local agencies and partnerships. Fast-loop activities in Holway were decided at the project meetings and could be implemented, and the impact observed, within weeks. The cycles have been characterised on the one hand by separate, sequential phases of action and research and on the other hand by action accompanied by, or indeed, infused with, processes of observation and data collection. The Triangle project's social event methodology built data collection into activities; its exercise and healthy eating activities were more amenable to more traditional forms of structured data collection, including surveys.

Inter-agency partnerships and negotiation for change

Action research depends on effective negotiation for change within partnerships drawn from researchers, service providers and other key community stakeholders. If action research into health inequalities and wider health determinants within communities demands collaborative action, collaboration demands active management (Huxham and Vangen, 2005). Partnerships flourish where the interests of individual partners, even if not declared, are met, where risks are avoided and where additional benefit is demonstrable. In establishing the conditions for action and research to be undertaken at all, in drawing out learning that informs and influences practice, and in seeking to sustain a capacity for responsiveness to community need and opportunity, the openness of action research challenges the way in which relationships have traditionally been maintained. As the discussion in Chapter Seven on evaluation and evidence also suggests, action research is not necessarily conducted according to common conceptions of neat and orderly observational research. Indeed, it may intrude significantly into decision making, not least if the processes by which priorities are set are a focus for action. Action research does not tend to report with a short final section on implications for action: it is more likely, rather, to seek a response from services, or assurances that the evidence produced will form a basis for deliberation within service agencies and with the community about how to respond. If the introduction of the action research projects into their local scenes was a first challenge, the common experience across SHARP has been that participatory, community-based action research requires a heavy, continuing commitment to maintenance of relationships and to negotiation with a wide range of participants and stakeholders.

There were differences in the experience and outcomes of these negotiations for change within partnerships in the various SHARP projects. Although the projects were proposed and then managed by local partnerships, as the projects started to define, concretely, what they would do and how they would operate a number found it difficult to effectively manage those partnerships. All found the lack of definitive control and authority in what Bryson and Crosby (1992) term a 'shared power' world. In this view, '... organisations and institutions must share objectives, activities, resources, power, or authority in order to achieve collective gains or minimize losses' (Bryson and Crosby, 1992, p xi). To achieve such a shared framework of understanding as the basis for collaborative capacity requires both leadership and planning, which Bryson and Crosby characterise as 'the organisation of hope' (see also Baum, 1997). In seeking to involve the range of organisations needed to understand and address the problems of health and wellbeing in the SHARP communities, many of the projects felt blocked, slowed up, or even undermined. Huxham and Vangen (2005) have noted that, in partnership working, events can conspire to slow progress and the experience is one of collaborative inertia rather than collaborative advantage. Key members of the team leave and knowledge, contacts, energy and impetus are lost; other priorities mean that agencies can neither make the time nor provide the resources to respond to SHARP's claims for attention. In some cases, a politics of responsibility (or indeed envy) has seemed to bite. The SHARP projects have been willing to critique current provision of services, to respond directly to community-based rather than professional diagnoses of need and to take risks; in contrast to established agencies and partnerships, they commanded uncommitted resource against a broad understanding of health and wellbeing. Local agencies have objected to projects' assertions of need and their advocacy for change in communities that are seen as already being in receipt of significant resources, especially since they would carry responsibility for meeting continuing revenue costs after the SHARP project ended. But part of the explanation for the variable pace of change can simply be found in the need to make sense of action – for the projects, to check that they are developing activities in an explicable and appropriate way.

For agencies working in particular jurisdictions and professional territories, the breadth of SHARP's approach to community health – health inequalities – took them to the margins of their 'legitimate interest'. SHARP's pathways started from strongly social conceptions of health, from what are termed the wider determinants – continuing education/lifelong learning; housing and transport; community disorder, stigma and reputation; social exclusion. Although there were a few notable exceptions, and although the actions proposed by communities and by the SHARP projects generally involved *small* investments of financial resources, the 'leap' may have seemed too great for others less immediately committed. SHARP projects reported two types of response: attempts by established agencies and partnerships to 'hijack' the project and to appropriate its resources through insistence that activities should focus on their set priorities; and marginalisation of tokenistic responses. The SHARP projects sought quickly to establish a position as equal partner and to maintain freedom to work on understanding what community-defined priorities might be rather than to respond immediately to established agendas. This could be joint work and yet the projects were aware that as partner agencies responded as they were invited to do, there was potential for tension – projects talked of their work being 'stretched' in unexpected ways. Each project sought ways of working through how different interests and priorities might be accommodated and to establish reference points that would help in determining what to do.

Plamping and colleagues (2000) reflect the weight of evidence in research into partnership working, that agreeing a broadly shared vision and goals is a crucial source of order in partnerships. Others, including Bardach (1998), Sullivan and Skelcher (2002) and Huxham and Vangen (2005), suggest that generalised goals may not be a sufficient spur to action and that it is possible to build strong partnership gradually through more limited points of commitment to joint action. The high levels of coordination, support and care, and resourcefulness and creativity in assembling the mix of resources required – meeting places, equipment and people – to make even small differences to communities that have very little has been notable. A middle ground between vision and specific actions may be the crucial area for debate in the SHARP partnerships, concerning the shared task, basic rules and principles of conduct, opportunities for action and agreements about 'priorities'. The question then is how partnership working at strategic, governance and operational (this last including practice and community) levels can be effectively linked to allow the project to maintain both direction and responsiveness (Sullivan and Skelcher, 2002; Sullivan et al, 2002).

In Wrexham, R2R weathered the immediate sceptical reaction of youth service professionals to the dedicated focus on girls and young women. Although the level of access to services and quality of experience of young women was known to be poor compared with that of young men, positive action was nevertheless seen as excluding young men unnecessarily and unfairly from its facilities. The support for the project at senior levels in the youth service was based on a clear mandate to redress the historical balance and R2R persisted with its strategy, despite initial concern and resistance from young men and youth service colleagues. The experience produced significant learning about the need for a strategy and for provision that effectively integrated provision rather than segregating services by gender, while ensuring that the old inequalities did not recur. In partnership settings where, by contrast to R2R, there was no clear authority to which to appeal to maintain the mandate and impetus for change, it was all too easy for change efforts to become delayed and stuck. Project leads had to be political fixers and diplomats as much as address what in many cases were complex and difficult research choices.

There is a literature that has examined influences on the variable experience, rate and pace of organisational change and innovation (Pettigrew et al, 1992; Newton et al, 2003). It distinguishes crudely between receptive and non-receptive, or resistant, contexts for change. A variety of factors are proposed as explaining why change takes hold quickly and surely in some localities and yet in others there is inertia or resistance. Coherence in policy, supportive general mandates and pressure, easily graspable purposes and goals, strong partnerships and networks and the presence of key people to lead change are some of the factors identified. Leadership in action research comes in various guises. First, and almost self-evidently, there is leadership in defining what the action research is about, the vision of knowledge to be gained from local action and inquiry and why it matters. Such intellectual leadership matters throughout. A second, crucial role, perhaps less often seen as leadership, involves holding the project together, acting as a point of reference, being there, acting as a buffer between different worlds. This role, set between the variety of groups – academic researchers, community activists and representatives of service organisations – is required to translate across languages and social worlds and to soak up the emotion that action research generates. A third form of leadership involves assembly work – pulling together materials and resources required to create the conditions for action and for research and holding them together. These acts of leadership sometimes require enormous courage and personal risk taking, but it is also important to recognise that action research also requires support from people who have the authority to say 'yea' or 'nay'. Local champions may often be outside of the project, but will nevertheless give resources and support to that project. This receptiveness also sometimes takes people to stick their head up above the parapet and say, 'I think this is good, even if we do not know if it is right, yet'.

Given the range of factors to be 'lined up', opportunities for change and innovation depend on repeated challenges to the status quo that are themselves based on 'a framework of shared understandings and practices, and which itself has to be revisable' (Pettigrew et al, 1992, p 275). They cite Unger's (1987) analysis that identifies 'the quality of direct relations among people, their capability to alter formative contexts of power …' as a key (see Pettigrew et al, 1992, p 275). Such an understanding of change – both why and how – has much in common with the character of collaborative action research. In particular, Pettigrew and colleagues (1992, p 289) ask 'how does one turn what is important into action?'. They suggest that two factors are crucial: the extent to which organisations are able and actively willing to look outwards and systematically to interpret and process information, and their ability to sustain both attention to change and the mobilisation of energy, or resource, for change.

Evidence from the SHARP projects suggests that the most receptive context for action research in/with communities seems to be found either where projects are committed to working with reasonably small groups of participants who perceive the benefits of such participation, or where they are based in or clearly aligned with a service-providing organisation requiring minimal external support to deliver the project. The latter situation was found in the Right 2 Respect project based in Wrexham youth service and discussed in the box opposite, as well as in the BeWEHL project managed by the University of Wales, Newport.

Right 2 Respect: embedding research into practice

Right 2 Respect was based in and led by Wrexham youth service: the community (of girls and young women) to which it related was defined in terms of the youth service's capacity to redress an historic failure to provide a service that provided equivalent development opportunities to those available to boys and young men. The similarity between action research and youth work was very important to the way in which the project was 'assimilated' into the wider youth work service. The project worker and head of youth service saw that action research made explicit "the cyclical framework of 'look, think, act, review' that good youth workers already follow":

> "Both are a trial and error approach that recognises no mistakes, just learning processes. So the philosophy fits."

That sense of confidence that action research 'fits' does not, however, mean that it is experienced as a stable, predictable or entirely 'knowable' process:

> "Things may not go how you expect, but they still work. Groups can mix well one week, and hate each other the next. And you don't always know why. Most things work – eventually."

R2R was firmly embedded in, and supported by, Wrexham youth service. Partnerships *at the operational level* initiated by the youth service and involving other services/agencies ensured that activities could be developed and provided in response to needs identified by the young women – car mechanics classes, for example.

The Barefoot project in Cardiff also responded directly to identified needs: there, women's access to the swimming pool was negotiated between the project, representatives of the community and the manager of a leisure centre as a specific activity. Here operational partnerships were established on the basis of a match between identified need and the established service interests of the partner organisations. In projects where the key partnerships were also about the governance of the project and about influence at the policy rather than service delivery level, and about change in the nature of services offered to communities, there are a different set of complexities, and indeed, resistances.

If we take partnership working to mean the development and maintenance of a positive, purposeful relationship between organisations

(Cropper, 1996; Huxham and Vangen, 2005), the range of barriers to effective partnership are now well recognised. These include differences in the way organisations work – their structures and the complexity of finding appropriate linkage points, differences in their organising and cultural practices, in their languages and their procedures, in their priorities for investment and action and in the recognition each is willing to afford the others as legitimate players in shaping and addressing the issues raised (Gray, 1989; Wistow and Hardy, 1991; Cropper, 1996).

Huxham and Vangen (2005) and other collaboration theorists (for example, Bardach, 1998; Sullivan and Skelcher, 2002) set out an agenda for partnership management, arguing that this involves awareness of the range of tensions that arise in:

- managing partnership aims, membership structures and boundaries;
- managing working processes and the contribution and allocation of resources through the partnership;
- building trust and accountability and managing power relations among partners;
- ensuring commitment, determination and compromise (or give and take) in undertaking partnership tasks.

The experiences of SHARP projects certainly confirm that there are significant issues to be addressed in drawing attention and shared commitment to issues of health inequality and the wider determinants of health. Aims, involvements and the shape of each project changed through the five years. The points at which greatest energy could be found varied over time. The original boards and steering groups, invaluable in setting the projects up, tended to lose their bite and, as Peck and colleagues (2004) suggest, at the extreme to become a ritual rather than a deliberative or governing forum. In particular, problems of non-receptivity are likely to be encountered when putative partners are not fully supportive of the work. In HYPP, for example, despite the Powys Health Alliance's pre-selection of certain initiatives (with their full agreement) as sites for HYPP's evaluation of services for young people, the project still encountered difficulties in establishing effective partnership relationships. Project staff tried to work with multiple agencies that have claimed different agendas and priorities that did not include enthusiasm for an action research approach. Triangle provides a similar case (see box opposite), although the context was to some extent doubly resistant, partly because of initial community scepticism about the value of engaging in research activity to achieve change, but also because the building of partnership relations with key agencies has been particularly challenging.

Triangle: realigning partnerships

Triangle's project was ambitious in proposing simultaneously to:

- support and evaluate capacity building and priority development in three Local Health Alliances (LHAs) by working with both 'core' and 'sub-groups' in these newly formed partnership organisations;
- draw on an action research approach to build the capacity of local communities to address *what they saw as* the broader determinants of health, through working with local people already engaged in health development activities in each LHA area;
- facilitate the development of partnership working between LHAs and communities.

On the face of it, the LHAs were ideal partners in Triangle's exploration of community. The three LHAs selected were perceived to be at very different stages of development with regard to their potential to provide an integrating network for a range of activities relating to health, social exclusion and economic development, and their ability to coordinate initiatives that promote sustainable health initiatives in socioeconomically deprived areas.

The project demonstrates the reflexive nature of an action research approach. One of the LHAs Triangle sought to work with was unwilling to accept the 'newcomer' except on its own terms – Triangle's resource would be welcome, but only as additional support in addressing the LHAs established priorities. At the LHA meetings with Triangle, although attendance was good, no single representative from any of the LHAs consistently attended all meetings. This lack of continuity of representation meant that Triangle team members needed to re-explain the purpose of the project at each meeting. LHA representatives seemed to find the concept of action research difficult to get to grips with and, at most meetings, questioned the purpose of the project and its value and relevance to them. The unpredictability inherent in, and the emergent nature of, the approach seemed to cause unease. Some LHA representatives also queried the 'performance management' and 'accountability' structures relating to Triangle. Others were dissatisfied with Triangle's proposed inclusive methods of working that aimed to share learning across the areas (by having the core team work across each of the LHAs and communities) and pressed instead for a 'dedicated' person to be allocated to them. Finding ways of "encouraging LHA members to see us as potential partners rather than interfering outsiders was challenging and time-consuming", as one Triangle representative put it. But equally, the LHA representatives found it difficult to play an advisory role rather than a management role on the Project Steering Group. When, realising 'it was difficult to establish any lasting and effective "bridging" connections between the alliances and local concerns – the languages, values and operational cultures of these two levels being rather too different to bridge easily' (Triangle, 2005), Triangle set about revising its organisational arrangements while reaffirming its purpose. The emphasis of the project shifted to the community level with a range of 'on-the-ground relations' with community development organisations and with reference groups to carry learning and insight into community issues from the project into what was a changing institutional framework.

Action research, insisting both on research and on responsive change on behalf of the specific communities to which the SHARP projects related, clearly proved a challenge for local agencies. Even with five years' duration and their origins in local partnership bids, the SHARP projects found it in many cases difficult to attract and then 'lock in' more complex institutional structures. In particular (and ironically since SHARP was about health inequalities), health service organisations and professionals proved most difficult to stimulate into even supporting roles within partnerships. The Holway project could not retain even the lone health professional who agreed to extend an outreach service on to the estate. In HYPP, the health promotion service could not sustain involvement. In other projects, the health partners were unable to bridge the long-term, strategic and rather abstract issue of health inequalities and the short-term, operational interventions that communities advised were needed or likely to sustain engagement. In many instances, activities were not drawn from what is a limited set of evidence-based health promotion interventions (Raphael, 2000; Speller et al, 1997), but rather were educational and social in character. Partnership steering groups proved to be useful mechanisms to share reports of activity and progress, but not to mobilise supportive action and resource against issues identified by communities. More specific operational linkages between projects, or their host organisations, and partner organisations led to new, although not always innovative, activities – community exercise classes; fruit and veg clubs; a film club.

Influence over policy and levels of commitment to communities has seemed easier to achieve in the less fragmentary organisational contexts where it is all too easy to feel marginalised or included only as a token, all the more so since, as we have illustrated, partnerships also tend to be unstable entities, subject to structural and personnel change.

Roles and responsibilities: the organisation of action research

Two ways of organising for action research emerged in the SHARP projects: specialisation of function and shared responsibilities. The pattern of investment in each project depended on the view it took of the relationship between action and research. First, and most commonly, projects designated the research function as the specialist responsibility of one or more key individuals – professionals with either research or project management and expertise relevant to health inequalities or the wider determinants of health. In the BeWEHL project, for example, while women participants were taught basic research skills and used those skills in undertaking their own research in the community, responsibility for the action research cycle (reflecting, planning, acting and reporting on the adult education process and its impacts) lay with the project coordinator. In HYPP, similarly, though young people also participated in projects that stimulated and held their interest – such as an 'asset-mapping' exercise using photography – the evaluation-focused action research was the responsibility of a university-appointed researcher. In other projects, too, a small number of people took responsibility for conducting most action research processes – choice of the foci for research, design of observation, data collection and recording, analysis and reporting. Second, and particularly in projects where community researchers were employed, projects formed in such a way that a much wider involvement in the action research process was possible – from the initiation of action specifically with research as well as community benefit in mind, to publication of findings. In these projects, the meaning of research was broad, including reflection on action and discursive modes of learning as well as more conventional forms of social science. Because of this democratising commitment, these projects required systems for development and support of the action research process and of the 'novice' action researcher. Mentoring between researcher and community counterparts thus complemented what in the end proved to be very limited formal training and education opportunities.

Action research with both organisations and communities needs to be conducted in a 'discreet' rather than 'overt' manner. An example of HYPP workers' 'discreet' approach to action research was where the team was trying to work with agencies that have different aims and agendas and, inevitably, limited resources. Action research in this context required the practitioners to work in a diplomatic manner and seek a compatibility of activity that was not necessarily easy to achieve. Conversely, action research with young people required sensitivity to their views and priorities to ensure that "they don't feel they're being used like guinea pigs". For example, young people were involved in conducting an 'asset-mapping' project in Llanwrtyd Wells, using digital cameras to record their perceptions of the community.

BeWEHL: ethical issues when the personal becomes a research finding

In BeWEHL, findings were a joint creation, held in co-ownership, and this had an impact on the production of 'evidence', both in relation to outcomes and, just as important, the context from which they were derived. Change was tracked through participants' 'personal statements' – taped conversations with the project coordinator, conducted yearly to provide a comparative record of the ways in which they perceive their own lives or attitudes to have changed as a result of their participation, perceived benefits to their children and family, and so on. These statements could be powerful rhetorical indicators of enhanced confidence and wellbeing (for example, "the project has helped me remember who I am – it's helped me find myself again"). The coordinator described their comments as "priceless, in terms of what they reveal". Yet these statements were, simultaneously, strangely devoid of context. Little sense emerged of the in-depth context of these women's lives in this particular community when compared, say, with their naturally occurring conversations with each other and in their informal discussions with the coordinator. One way of providing richly contextualised evidence of change that had occurred through community participation in action research is to present 'stories' – case studies in a detailed narrative form. Although BeWEHL project leaders endorsed this approach, its implementation was problematic for the project coordinator and participants. Some women made it clear to project staff that key aspects of their 'stories' were not only personal but should remain private. While project staff are bound to honour this ethical obligation to confidentiality, it means that some elements of the context within which the project worked were difficult to report. Negotiating consent was a delicate process, in part to explain what use in a report would entail and what choices were to be made. However, the process of seeking consent was not solely about gaining the right to draw on personal data gained through the action research process. Participants may have been keen to engage in potentially damaging self-exposure, placing their research project firmly in the context of difficulties experienced in their own lives. This was an area of anxiety for project staff who valued the richness of the data thus provided but were also concerned that participants' relative research inexperience, at this stage, meant that their understanding of the longer-term implications of public autobiographical disclosure was inevitably limited.

Conclusion

In their discussion of the experimenting society, Donald Campbell and Jean Russo (1999) argue that such a society would be committed to a variety of values, which they set out as an ideology: 'It would be an active society, preferring exploratory innovation to inaction.... It will be committed to *action research*, to action as research rather than research as a postponement of action' (p 13, emphasis in original). It would be honest, self-critical, and committed to learning and to science in what Campbell and Russo describe as the fullest sense of the word 'scientific', in which evidence informs design of interventions, but in which there is also the strongest commitment to understanding the effects and effectiveness of those interventions and to challenge and accountability. Finally, they conclude by arguing that such a society would also be decentralising, encouraging of popular participation and responsive to collective expressions of interest, need and preference. Against these values, the SHARP projects score highly, we believe. They reveal that the vision of careful, principled innovation is both one to which many aspire and one that can be achieved, although the institutionalisation of these values in practice takes sustained effort and care, against other prevailing institutional norms – bureaucracy, risk aversion, control and narrowed senses of accountability. Creating systems, indeed communities, of intelligent action and learning requires a collaborative capacity around what we have termed action research partnerships, and we have suggested some characteristics of that capacity. At its heart are different forms of leadership, including the intellectual drive for intelligent change. Chapter Seven reports on use of the idea of articulate theories of change as a way of opening planned action to scrutiny, debate and testing. Action research demands attention to the basis for intervention, not least because of the duty to monitor and evaluate how action bites. In reflecting on their experience of evaluating Health Action Zones in England, Barnes and colleagues (2005, p 188) report:

> We began with high expectations about the use of theory-based evaluation in general and theories of change in particular. For a whole series of reasons ... this did not materialize in the way that we had originally hoped. Our expectation that local actors could be persuaded to articulate and adhere to sophisticated strategies for change contained a large element of wishful thinking. There is also a real sense in which the approach assumes too much of a linear view of the world, which is at odds with the continuous process of interaction and adjustment to changing circumstances experienced by local actors. But ... it can and does help local planning.... Our experience is that it is easier for practitioners to accommodate it at programme or project level, whereas attempting to create a Theory of Change at strategic level is much more demanding.... In addition, the approach might have a different and possibly equally valuable contribution to building the evidence base for effective social change.

By contrast with the evaluation of Health Action Zones, the experience in SHARP was that theories of change at both strategic and practice levels were held, were capable of articulation and of being shared, and were monitored and changed as a consequence of experience. The idea of a 'theory' was not necessarily helpful in practice – given its scientific connotation, it could seem daunting to action researchers bound up in the detail of particular situations; and the sense that it might be singular rather than layered and plural was also initially disconcerting. Theories of intervention and change inevitably proved to be complex, although there was likely to be one (or more) core idea that was being tried and tested. In Chapter Seven, Sandra Carlisle and colleagues reflect further on the ways in which the metaphor of a theory of change can be helpful in understanding the relationship between action, research and evaluation.

In research and in evaluation, it is never possible to collect all the data you want. Focused data collection, and focused discussions about particular ideas and propositions are important, but openness to data that emerge is also crucial: a theory is a way of seeing, but also of not seeing. Whether or not outcomes will be realised and observed in the project's lifetime will depend on the project's theory of change, on the sharpness of the mechanisms and on the lead time, or lag, before outcomes become visible in the relevant context. Learning about these is itself a research (and action-relevant) outcome.

Lewin (1948) emphasised that the research data (in his case, concerned with understanding the kinds of change his workshops produced) would be complex and difficult to keep hold of (see also Huxham and Eden, 1996). The need to design methods for recording ill-structured data was therefore important; focus on relationship between perception and action was also important.

In getting health action research projects up, running and on their way in some orderly way, there are some practical challenges. Action research can seem a precarious task, requiring skill in coordinating the worlds of research, policy, community, the professions and public agencies (Dawson, 1997). One of the strengths of the SHARP programme has been its determination to fuse action and inquiry in a variety of ways, and in its attempts to test whether community-articulated needs, collected in a rigorous and credible way, will be listened to, and whether statutory, voluntary and community-based organisations will be able to respond.

References

Balloch, S. and Taylor, M. (eds) (2001) *Partnership Working: Policy and Practice*, Bristol: The Policy Press.

Balogh, R., Markwell, S. and Watson, J. (2004) *Action Research Resource Pack*, Cardiff: Welsh Assembly Government.

Bardach, E. (1998) *Getting Agencies to Work Together: The Practice and Theory of Managerial Craftsmanship*, Washington, DC: Brookings Institution Press.

Barnes, M., Bauld, L., Benzeval, M., Mackenzie, M., Sullivan, H. and Judge, K. (2005) *Health Action Zones: Partnerships for Health Equity*, London: Routledge.

Baum, H.S. (1997) *The Organization of Hope: Communities Planning Themselves*, Albany, NY: State University of New York.

Benington, J. (1974) 'Strategies for change at the local level: some reflections', in D. Jones and M. Mayo (eds) *Community Work 1*, London: Routledge and Kegan Paul, pp 260-77.

Benington, J. (1997) 'Risk and reciprocity: local governance rooted within civil society', in A. Coulson (ed) *Trust and Contracts: Relationships in Local Government, Health and Public Services*, Bristol: The Policy Press, pp 227-42.

Boutilier, M., Mason, R. and Rootman, I. (1997) 'Community action and reflective practice in health promotion research', *Health Promotion International*, vol 12, pp 69-78.

Bryson, J.M. and Crosby, B.C. (1992) *Leadership for the Common Good: Tackling Public Problems in a Shared-power World*, San Francisco, CA: Jossey Bass.

Burnes, B. (2004) 'Kurt Lewin and the planned approach to change: a re-appraisal', *Journal of Management Studies*, vol 41, pp 977-1002.

Campbell, D.T. and Russo, M.J. (1999) *Social Experimentation*, Thousand Oaks, CA: Sage Publication.

Cassell, C. and Johnson, P. (2006) 'Action Research: explaining the diversity', *Human Relations*, vol 59, pp 783-814.

Chandler, D. and Torbert, B. (2003) 'Transforming inquiry and action: interweaving 27 flavors of action research', *Action Research,* vol 1, pp 133-52.

Cropper, S.A. (1996) 'Collaborative working and the issue of sustainability', in C.S. Huxham (ed) *Creating Collaborative Advantage*, London: Sage Publications, pp 80-100.

Dawson, S. (1997) 'Inhabiting different worlds: how can research relate to practice?', *Quality in Health Care*, vol 6, pp 177-8.

Dick, B. (1999) 'What is action research?', www.scu.edu.au/schools/gcm/ar/whatisar.html

Eden, C. and Huxham, C. (1996) 'Action research for the study of organizations', in S. Clegg, C. Hardy and W. Nord (eds) *Handbook of Organizational Studies*, London: Sage Publications.

Gittel, R. and Vidal, A. (1998) *Community Organizing: Building Social Capital as a Development Strategy*, Thousand Oaks, CA: Sage Publications.

Gray, B. (1989) *Collaborating*, San Francisco, CA: Jossey Bass.

Hammersley, M. (1999) *Taking Sides in Social Research: Essays on Partisanship and Bias in Social Enquiry*, London: Routledge.

Hart, E. and Bond, M. (1995) *Action Research for Health and Social Care*, Buckingham: Open University Press.

Heller, F. (1993) 'Another look at action research', *Human Relations*, vol 46, no 10, pp 1235-42.

Huxham, C.S. and Eden, C. (1996) 'Action research for the study of organizations', in S. Clegg, C. Hardy and W. Nord (eds) *The Handbook of Organizational Studies*, London: Sage Publications, pp 526-42.

Huxham, C.S. and Vangen, S. (2003) 'Researching organizational practice through action research: case studies and design choices', *Organizational Research Methods*, vol 6, pp 383-403.

Huxham, C.S. and Vangen, S. (2005) *Managing to Collaborate: The Theory and Practice of Collaborative Advantage*, London: Routledge.

Kemmis, S. (2001) 'Exploring the relevance of critical theory for action research', in P. Reason and H. Bradbury (eds) *Handbook of Action Research: Participative Enquiry and Practice*, London: Sage Publications.

Lewin, K. (1948) 'Action research and minority problems', in K. Lewin and G.W. Lewin (eds) *Resolving Social Conflicts*, London: Souvenir Press, pp 201-16.

Marris, P. and Rein, M. (1967) *Dilemmas of Social Reform*, London: Routledge.

Mayo, M. (1974) 'Strategies for change: two critiques', in D. Jones and M. Mayo (eds) *Community Work 1*, London: Routledge and Kegan Paul, pp 241-4.

Newton, J., Graham J., McLoughlin, K. and Moore, A. (2003) 'Receptivity to change in a general medical practice', *British Journal of Management*, vol 14, pp 143-53.

Peck, E., 6, P., Gulliver, P. and Towell, D. (2004) 'Why do we keep on meeting like this? The board as ritual in health and social care', *Health Services Management Research*, vol 17, pp 100-9.

Pettigrew, A., Ferlie, E. and McKee, L. (1992) *Shaping Strategic Change*, London: Sage Publications.

Plamping, D., Gordon, P. and Pratt, J. (2000) 'Modernising the NHS: practical partnerships for health and local authorities', *British Medical Journal*, vol 320, pp 1723-5.

Raphael, D. (2000) 'The question of evidence in health promotion', *Health Promotion International*, vol 15, no 4, pp 355-67.

Rapoport, R. (1970) 'Three dilemmas in action research', *Human Relations*, vol 23, no 6, pp 499-513.

Reason, P. (1994) 'Three approaches to participative enquiry', in N. Denzin and Y. Lincoln (eds) *Handbook of Qualitative Research*, London: Sage Publications.

Reason, P. and Bradbury, H. (2001) (eds) *Handbook of Action Research: Participative Enquiry and Practice*, London: Sage Publications.

Rein, M. (1976) *Social Science and Public Policy*, Harmondsworth: Penguin.

Sandberg, R. (1985) 'Socio-technical design, trade union strategies and action research', in E. Mumford, R. Hirschheim, G. Fitzgerald and T. Wood-Harper (eds) *Research Methods in Information Systems*, Amsterdam: North-Holland-Elsevier Science, pp 79-92.

Speller, V., Learmouth, A. and Harrison, D. (1997) 'The search for evidence of effective health promotion', *British Medical Journal*, vol 315, pp 361-3.

Stringer, E. (1996) *Action Research: A handbook for Practitioners*, Thousand Oaks, CA: Sage Publications.

Sullivan, H. and Skelcher, C. (2002) *Working across Boundaries: Collaboration in Public Services*, Basingstoke: Palgrave.

Sullivan, H., Barnes, M. and Matka, E. (2002) 'Building collaborative capacity through "theories of change": early lessons from the evaluation of Health Action Zones in England', *Evaluation*, vol 8, pp 205-26

Susman, G.I. (1983) 'Action research: a sociotechnical systems perspective', in G. Morgan (ed) *Beyond Method*, London: Sage Publications.

Trevillion, S. (1999) *Networking and Community Partnership* (2nd edn), Aldershot: Arena.

Triangle (2005) *Phase 2 Report*, Cardiff: School of Social Sciences, University of Wales.

Waterman, H., Tillen, D., Dickson, R. and de Koning, K. (2001) 'Action research: a systematic review and guidance for assessment', *Health Technology Assessment*, vol 5, no 23.

Whitelaw, S., Beattie, A., Balogh, R. and Watson, J. (2003) *A Review of the Nature of Action Research*, Cardiff: Welsh Assembly Government.

Whyte, W.F. (ed) (1991) *Participatory Action Research*, London: Sage Publications.

Winter, R. and Munn-Giddings, C. (2001) *A Handbook for Action Research in Health and Social Care*, London: Routledge.

Wistow, G. and Hardy, B. (1991) 'Joint management in community care', *Journal of Management in Medicine*, vol 5, pp 44-8.

FIVE

Engaging with communities

Bronwen Bermingham and Alison Porter

Introduction

This chapter sets out learning from the Sustainable Health Action Research Programme (SHARP) about the character of communities, strategies for the development of relationships with communities, and the difficulties encountered in those relationships. It also considers the outcomes – more and less tangible – that may survive as meaningful resources for continuing community–agency relations. We consider community engagement as a continuing process, and one in which initial engagement and re-engagement offer particular challenges to both communities and to the SHARP partnerships.

Engagement of the SHARP projects with the communities within which they were working has been a fundamental criterion of their success. There are two reasons for this. First, the projects needed to engage with communities in order to give themselves academic credibility: it is no good basing a project on what communities perceive as their own health needs if you cannot demonstrate that community members themselves have defined and articulated those needs. Second, by its very nature, action research is based on engagement and cannot function without it. Engagement with communities is necessary both to identify needs but also to convert understandings of needs into interventions, resources and practices that may bring about change.

The terms 'engagement', 'involvement' and 'participation' are all used to discuss the processes by which organisations and their users, or the broader community, can work together on the planning, design, delivery and monitoring of services. These processes are seen as essential to ensuring that public services are appropriate in nature and delivered in an appropriate way; and community involvement, community strategies and community leadership have become key building blocks of New Labour's approach to public policy and public service delivery. The Health Development Agency (HDA) has defined the 'new' public health agenda as focusing on community-based frameworks to affect the underlying determinants of health inequalities (Rogers and Robinson,

2004), while the Department of Health has commissioned the Nuffield Institute for Health to produce a series of guides to community involvement for providers of health and social care in England (Emmel, 2004; Emmel and Conn, 2004). However, as was pointed out in work for the Audit Commission, the concept of community involvement is both slippery and potentially troublemaking:

> Community and neighbourhood involvement ... remains a vague concept and outcomes are ill-defined. Finding a satisfactory description of what it is and why it is done involves an exploration of all the ways in which communities are involved in public affairs. (Smyth, 2001, p 1)

While 'involvement' is a concept that encompasses these broad themes of power and control, the term 'engagement' may be thought of as referring more specifically to the actual process of interaction between a community and, in this case, a SHARP project. It implies reciprocity: the project engages with the community and the community engages with the project, a model that is unfamiliar to traditional social research (see Chapter Seven). It also emphasises the fact that there is a process going on that may change through time, and that requires action, management and maintenance. For this reason, 'engagement' has been chosen as the theme of this chapter.

Processes of engagement work in more than one direction, since they are about how groups who may have very different starting points, expectations and agendas meet and interact. This chapter will consider the extent to which communities engaged with the various SHARP projects, and the extent to which this was on the projects' terms. It will also consider how successful projects were at engaging with communities on communities' own terms – which may, of course, be many different sets of terms according to the layering and grouping within a community. Within the SHARP programme, there was also a third set of processes in operation – that concerned with smoothing the mutual engagement of communities and service providers. The skill with which SHARP projects oiled the wheels of these sometimes troubled relationships is considered in more detail in Chapter Eight.

The experience of all the projects within SHARP is at odds with unitary conceptions of community, community leadership and voice, and we reflect on how a variety of relationships with communities can be established and maintained. We explore the ways in which communities can be understood as stratified, sometimes deeply, and discuss strategies to enable not only initial contact to take place, but also the deepening of engagement. The roles of community members and 'accepted outsiders' in promoting engagement are central to the discussion of strategies for engagement. Many of the SHARP communities have been weakly linked to service agencies, have had poor experiences of consultation and few community resources; trust in statutory agencies is commonly low.

The chapter concludes with a discussion of how progress in engagement can be judged, considers ways in which community capacity becomes defined and articulated, and explores the release of power to communities and the management of risk by both communities and agencies in that process. It examines how engagement and the depth of engagement is acknowledged, recorded and experienced; and it considers the extent to which this is an integral part of evaluating the success and impact of a project or programme, and the extent to which it might be considered as a separate process.

The nature of communities

Geographical communities and communities of interest

If the process of engagement takes place between the project and the community, the obvious question is: what is the community? Should it be considered in this context as a place, a set of people with common interest, a mode of activity or as a mechanism for giving collective legitimacy to individual perspectives? At a pragmatic level, should the focus for defining a 'community' be a set of shared problems that can provide a focus for shared action? In this case, what are the implications of identifying a community by a sense of shared problems or need?

Among those working in the field of community initiatives for health improvement, there is little agreement about what a community is (Jewkes and Murcott, 1996; Emmel and Conn, 2004; Barnes et al, 2007). Yet definition of the community (or communities) is needed not just for conceptual clarity but also for practical reasons. The SHARP projects have needed to define the communities with which they would be working in order to target their activities, to limit the scale of their work, and to give them some framework against which they can measure what they have achieved. Inevitably, the definitions applied were diverse.

The seven projects can be broadly divided into two types: communities of identity and communities of place (Carlisle et al, 2004). 'Communities of identity' are those where members are perceived to have common attributes or characteristics, and may be assumed to have some degree of common outlook or experience. 'Communities of place' are identified with a particular neighbourhood or location;

this sounds straightforward, but in fact raises all sorts of questions about the size of area people identify with, diversity or cohesion within a geographical area, and the role of place itself in promoting or harming health. Table 5.1, taken from the overarching evaluation, shows how the SHARP projects may be clustered both in terms of type of community with which they were working, and in terms of how intensive or extensive were the processes of engagement that took place with those communities.

Table 5.1: SHARP project clusters

	Communities of place	Communities of identity
Intensively focused action research	Holway House project	BeWEHL HYPP R2R
Extensively focused action research	Pembrokeshire SHARP Triangle project	'Barefoot' Health Workers project

Source: Carlisle et al (2004)

The definitions of 'community of place' and 'community of identity' are not absolutely mutually exclusive. For example, Barefoot, while working within specific city wards, also stated the precise minority ethnic groups with which it would engage. BeWEHL (Bettws Women's Education, Health and Lifestyle) defined its community as being women from the Bettws estate in Newport; this was both a community of place and a community of presumed shared interest and outlook. The BeWEHL project reveals another complexity, in that there were two different types or levels of engagement taking place with two differently targeted communities. One level of engagement was with the relatively small group of socially isolated women who took part in adult education courses. These women then acted as the bridge to another level of engagement with the wider community, through research projects into community health needs.

How communities get to be defined

Definitions of community do not just exist; they have to be created by someone and, to an extent, maintained and reinforced in a continuous process. In some cases, the selection of the community of interest was part of the development of a research question. The HYPP (Health of Young People in Powys) project, for example, wanted to investigate what difference it makes to work with different types of community within the population of young people in Powys. 'Community' was defined by HYPP in a number of different ways: in the OASIS initiative, it was about the school community, while in Llanwrtyd Wells it was a community of young people, and in the New Deal project it was the community of service users.

In some cases, the definition of the targeted community was refined and developed during the course of the project. Right 2 Respect, for example, worked in its first phase with just one group of young women, from one school. The second phase of the project broadened this to six more groups, with a wider age range and from different communities, not just deprived areas. At the same time, as the project progressed, the interests of young men became evident and their specific needs, including, by implication, their need for engagement, were acknowledged by the project.

Definitions of community created and used by community members may be very different from those that originate with outsiders, such as health development workers (Cohen, 1985; Jewkes and Murcott, 1996). The process of definition of communities can lead to tensions when externally defined identities are not readily accepted by community members. Some definitions, such as 'an area of deprivation', carry negative connotations that may cause distress or embarrassment, or simply be rejected by those living there (Popay et al, 2003). Awareness of these issues was apparent from many comments made by project workers working closely with the communities. For example, BeWEHL's workers were reported in the overarching evaluation as being keenly aware that conventional ways of representing and speaking about people living in positions of socioeconomic disadvantage could be inappropriate and unworkable. They viewed the term 'socially isolated' as meaningless, and said that community members found the term 'socially excluded' offensive (Carlisle et al, 2004).

The rural community of Llanychaer in north Pembrokeshire was part of the SHARP Pembrokeshire project. Here, as in BeWEHL, there was resistance from community members, in this case to being incorporated into what they saw as an 'experiment', unsuited to this relatively prosperous location. Confident and articulate members of the Llanychaer local forum, set up as part of the project, were willing and able to question – with some success – the terms of the 'experiment' in which they were being asked to participate. The forum also successfully challenged the partnership's initial ideas of how 'the community' should be defined, requiring it to broaden its original research boundaries. This resistance to the process of definition evolved into an active and productive role for the forum in refining the plans for the project's engagement with the wider community (Carlisle et al, 2004).

Layers within communities

Guidance from the UK government about community involvement and engagement is largely based on an implicit assumption that communities have a solidarity that can be expressed as a single voice (ODPM, 2003), with shared 'views', 'wants' and 'needs' (Wilmott and Thomas, 1984). Jewkes and Murcott (1996), in their work on community participation in health promotion, have explored how the metaphor of community as person is used, identifying the community as an entity with the capacity to think and make decisions, and with its own expertise and agenda.

By contrast, the SHARP experience highlighted the layers and multiple networks, and the fractures and feuds within communities. The engagement process in the SHARP programme took place on many different layers, with different players establishing their own particular forms of engagement with different layers or strata within the different targeted communities. Some projects found that their original ambitions of engaging with a whole community were unrealistic, and that more success came when they targeted their attentions on groups within a community. Importantly, these smaller groups were not interpreted as 'representing' the community as a whole; instead, the scale of both action and research was adjusted to reflect the engagement.

Within any community, some groups may be more ready to engage than others. The Barefoot project, for example, found that, to a large extent, the route into communities was through the women. They tended to be highly motivated by a desire for advancement and jobs and, indirectly, for a more independent position within their own communities. In addition, the Women in Action swimming project, jointly initiated by Barefoot and Triangle, gave the women an opportunity to socialise and exercise with female members of their families. Meanwhile, the Holway project struggled to engage a small core of hard-to-reach unemployed men. But there was some success – 10 of the men became involved in a summer Youth Challenge, and two of these subsequently went on to education and training.

Some of the SHARP projects reported that they were aware of the ways in which techniques for engagement might produce a natural bias, which will have implications for any information gathered from them. For example, the Triangle project set up a consultation activity that involved handing out free kettles, and found that it brought in a disproportionate number of middle-aged and older people, particularly women. The activity was used as a social event within which basic data could be collected about community views, and these indicated considerable anxiety about the behaviour of children and young people that may have been a reflection of inter-generational distance and conflict.

The Holway project involved working in a single, tightly bounded estate, which might be thought to present a straightforward opportunity for engagement with a relatively uniform community. In fact, the project team found that the Holway estate had different 'zones', some of which were seen as more problematic than others. In addition, some resentment was expressed by people within the estate who felt that too much was being done by SHARP for 'less deserving' people. For example, there were conflicts over the use of the community hall – the bingo club was unwilling to give up bookings to allow use by the summer youth project. Criticism was also levelled by some community members against the Holway project because it was seen to be doing too little for implicitly 'deserving' older people.

In many ways, the task of working with complex communities was easier for those SHARP projects that worked with communities that were more clearly divided geographically as well as in social or economic terms. Both the Pembrokeshire and the Triangle projects, for example, worked with three communities, geographically isolated from one another, and with quite distinct characteristics and local cultures. Both projects handled this by managing their respective interventions in three quite distinct parts, Triangle going so far as to have three, locally recruited, project workers, one for each area. In this way, processes of research and action were tailor-made for the three different communities within each project.

Processes of engagement
Building on existing links

To a greater or lesser degree, all of the projects built on existing links and partnerships to help in the task of bringing about engagement. The overarching evaluation team observed that engagement was most effective where groundwork had already been done: links made, trust established and support structures put in place for the sometimes fragile relationships established through the SHARP projects' processes of engagement. By building on existing links, the projects gained a number of benefits. The most straightforward was where existing organisations provided a structure within which the action and the research could take place. This is one aspect of the partnership work discussed in Chapter Four. In some cases, the existing organisations provided more than just a framework: the HYPP project, for example, used existing structures such as a drop-in information service in a school and a Healthy Communities project in Llanwrtyd Wells as the basis of the 'action' component of the action research. In the Holway project, the existing community-based activity in the area, such as a youth club, community workers and so on, provided more of a backdrop to the SHARP work. It also may have helped to introduce residents to the idea of community-based activity of a sort that was strikingly lacking in some other locations, such as the rural Pembrokeshire site of Llanychaer, or among the Yemeni community with which Barefoot was working in Cardiff.

An additional benefit to building on existing links was seen where groundwork had already begun in terms of identifying community needs. For example, even before the SHARP project began, some residents of the Holway project were active in identifying goals on which they wanted action – fly-tipping, speeding, antisocial behaviour and so on. The SHARP project came into a receptive environment, and was able to act as a catalyst for change, in this case the installation of CCTV.

Relationships with organisations already working in a community may not be straightforward, however. One of the communities with which Barefoot was working, for example, already had a strong voluntary sector women's organisation. Developing work with this community meant that the SHARP project worker had to handle some difficult power issues with the group. A relationship that suited both the group and the project was established when a joint exercise class was set up, with publicity material acknowledging the input of both organisations as equal partners.

Spaces of engagement

Engagement does not take place in the abstract, but is acted out in the real world. Thinking about what might be called the spaces of engagement brings a focus to the actual processes that take place. Spaces of engagement may be read as territory – theirs, yours or ours – and the various ways in which community members respond to those spaces may facilitate or block engagement. On a small scale, a space of engagement may be somewhere such as Holway House (described in the box opposite) where community members could come without feeling alienated. On a larger scale, the idea of spaces of engagement brings a focus to the issue of how neighbourhoods are defined and 'owned' by the people who live in them, and where the geographical boundaries of a neighbourhood are drawn. People's willingness to engage may be directly affected by their sense of connectedness with the place where they live.

The Holway house: whose territory?

For Holway, the house was the key feature of the project work, with the stated aim of improving residents' quality of life and equalising access for all to the basic prerequisites of health. The local democratic partnership has succeeded in establishing the house as the contact point for the community by a number of service providers such as the local college, which offers residents both recreational and vocational courses. The Holway house was hugely important as a location for both formal and casual meetings. About 20 adults and children would drop in to eat at the house, and some made sandwiches there. All the food in the house was 'healthy', with no crisps or biscuits. People were suspicious at first, but seemed to grow to like it. The house was also the location for the homework club – a popular venue for young people, where relations were less formal than in school. The club included pupils who had been excluded from school. The house contained computers that were used by the homework club, by residents learning IT, and by residents producing a community newsletter.

While those who attended the Holway house appeared to feel a sense of 'belonging' in the space, they were a minority of the population of the estate. There was a degree of polarisation between those residents who used the house and those who used other facilities such as the community centre.

The Holway project was unusual in being so tightly focused on one intervention, in one place. Other projects were much more diverse in terms of their spaces of engagement, but still had experience of creating spaces where community members would feel a sense of belonging.

Right 2 Respect went out to six diverse communities and found spaces of engagement in each. For example, in Glyn Ceiriog (a rural community) the group met in the community centre and, when this was unavailable, in the local pub. Project workers reported feeling accepted and supported by the people who managed these spaces. In another Right 2 Respect location, the semi-rural community of Gresford, the young women designed and fitted out their own room in a youth centre, for use for meetings, peer support and quiet discussion. They chose décor and furnishings to create the right kind of atmosphere. In Llay (a suburb of Wrexham), Right 2 Respect struggled when the only available venue was a dilapidated youth centre, and even more so once that was demolished. But when, in its place, was built a brand new lifelong learning centre the project really took off – especially as the centre manager was very supportive.

Where suitable spaces were lacking, engagement processes were hampered. Barefoot project workers in Cardiff's Butetown tried to avoid engaging community members in private spaces such as people's homes, preferring to find places that were more neutral and less intrusive, without any risks to safety. But many of the more public meeting spaces in the area were seen as partisan or unacceptable: many Muslim people were reluctant to go into church halls, for example. There were similar issues in Riverside, where Barefoot worked with Triangle to support the Women in Action group: at a community planning event, Women in Action members talked of their dream of a building for their needs, with a hall, kitchen, prayer room and crèche. It would be a space they could call their own that would validate the group's existence.

Changing engagement over time

The engagement of a community in action research is not a one-off event, but a dynamic process that has to be maintained throughout the life of the projects. It can be broken down into four broad stages – initial engagement, on-going engagement, re-engagement and disengagement. At each of these stages, which do not necessarily unfold in a simply linear fashion, engagement may be based on a different mix of people, and different levels of trust, enthusiasm, suspicion and conflict. At the same time, the role of individuals involved in the process may evolve and develop.

All the projects found that building relationships of trust with communities was a slow process that had to take place at the start of the involvement before any overt action research activities could take place. The experience of the Triangle project, described in the box opposite, provides another illustration of how work was designed to allow for this.

Triangle: softly, softly

The Triangle project began by taking a slow, gentle and reactive approach to the process of engagement. A good deal of time was spent in the early stages just meeting and listening to local people in order to gain an understanding not only of the most pressing wellbeing issues, but also of the cultural and social norms that influenced these views and people's responses to them. It seemed at first as if the project were lacking in direction and action, but in retrospect this cautious start was critical to ensuring that when the first tentative actions were encouraged they resonated with local people who then voluntarily participated. At this stage, overt research was kept low-key and at times almost imperceptible, while emphasis was placed on responding practically and genuinely to locally perceived needs. This established action research as 'reciprocal' in nature rather than of the orthodox 'extractive' variety was something that made it much more acceptable and meaningful to those who became involved in the Triangle project.

This approach to contacting and networking with local people, and of raising awareness of local facilities, was developed very much through 'word of mouth'. As part of the project, a workshop bringing together a range of people active in the community was used to draft a 'toolkit' for developing a word-of-mouth network.

Transition through the phases of engagement did not always go at the pace that might have been expected. In Pembrokeshire, the project found that initial engagement was established with relative ease. However, in the absence of external investment or resources, community groups lacked the capacity and confidence to take the work further, and the credibility of the project in the wider community was undermined by local experiences of little or no change. In the rural community, by contrast, the Pembrokeshire project struggled to make the initial engagement, but once this was established, there was a remarkable degree of local commitment to action research. Holway project workers observed a change over time in the nature of people's engagement, in that they became more analytical. They also observed how residents' capacity to participate in the formal structures of engagement – their ability to manage orderly meetings and so on – developed during the course of the project.

At an individual level, some people involved with the SHARP projects went through substantial changes in the nature of their engagement as part of a personal progress of change of role and change of relationship with the project. In Right 2 Respect, young people in the Brynteg group became so engaged with the project that they took part in interviews for new youth workers joining the team. In the Barefoot project, one key community member who started out as a member of the women's swimming initiative also became a regular catering supplier to the project. She experienced a change of relationship from receiving assistance, both in capacity and financial terms, to negotiating a professional fee for a service provided to the organisation. This indicates a power shift in the relationship from one of initial dependence to one of greater equality.

Another example of this is provided by the BeWEHL project. The project, which worked with 160 women over five years, aimed to increase health and confidence in women who would be considered excluded. The initial intake of students 'graduated' from their involvement in the Making a Difference volunteering programme to studentship as part of Further Education Development. With the move from one group to another, the relationship between the members and the project changed.

The nature of engagement between project and community can be affected by changes in the individual people involved. The Right 2 Respect groups experienced turnover as some young people grew out of them and new, younger girls joined. These changes seemed to be fairly smooth. By contrast, changes in staff members resulted in serious disruption to engagement in a number of projects, including Barefoot. Two community researchers departed during the lifetime of the project, leaving vacancies that took many months to fill. This resulted in loss of engagement and a need to re-engage after the recruitment of the new community researchers.

Barriers and motivations to engagement
Perspectives and expectations

Engagement may be helped or, more likely, hindered by the perspectives and expectations of any of the parties involved. The very word 'health' proved off-putting in some contexts. Some – though not all – projects found that presenting 'health' as the theme of the projects could actually be counter-productive. Instead, it needed to be viewed in terms of broader wellbeing and quality of life, since that is how most people see the issue.

More than one of the SHARP projects discovered how names and titles can saddle projects with unexpected baggage, which in turn inhibits engagement. Though most local people seemed happy with the title 'Right 2 Respect', a few felt it conveyed a threatening image, one that could be read as un-female or anti-male. The title of the Barefoot project was chosen to reflect a concept from international development work, where 'barefoot' describes skilled health workers 'of the people'. However, many people, particularly in the Somali and Yemeni communities, found the expression 'barefoot' offensive, since they felt it implied that it was they who were barefoot, poor and unsophisticated. Project workers with these communities quietly dropped the name in their dealings with the community, and described the project instead as the Health Promotion project.

Differences in perspectives and expectations can work in both directions, and there are examples of academics' lack of understanding of community members' agendas, as well as the other way round. The example from Pembrokeshire, in the box below, illustrates one of the risks to the engagement processes posed by interaction between people with widely different perspectives.

Pembrokeshire: a gap in understanding

As part of their training in the research process, the community researchers in the Pembrokeshire SHARP project took part in a practice interviewing exercise. The academic trainer presented them with one of the questions to be used in the research: 'What do you like about living here?'. In the discussion of the responses, the community researchers brought in their personal experiences to reflect on what was being talked about. The trainer observed that people's answers were quite fatalistic: 'What do you like about living here?' – "Well, I've always lived here". She could see something interesting in that response – people weren't answering the question, they were saying, 'What's the point of answering the question?'.

But the community researchers challenged this interpretation: "But that's the right answer…. Because we all live here, we've always lived here and we don't have a choice about going anywhere else". They became quite personally involved and quite defensive. The project's main action researcher, a full-time member of staff, reported:

> "I nearly lost them on that day. They all came away saying, 'I'm not doing that again – that was hopeless!'"

As much as possible, the projects made efforts to be sensitive to the perspective of community members in terms of the barriers they were experiencing to taking part in project activities. Wherever possible, these were addressed by structuring activities in a way that minimised those barriers. For example, barriers may be presented by other demands on the time of potential participants. In Right 2 Respect, a lot of the young women were responsible for babysitting younger siblings, as parents worked in the evenings, or they had evening jobs themselves. Meetings were therefore held at teatime – straight after school or college. Similarly, in BeWEHL, childcare was one of the biggest barriers to engagement, particularly for women who were on low incomes but were not eligible for state benefits. In the Barefoot project, there were different issues: meetings were held during the daytime at weekends, to allow people who worked in the restaurant trade to attend. However, people will choose what activities they are interested in taking part in. In both Holway and Pembrokeshire, for example, project workers struggled to involve community members in preparing written reports.

Research fatigue and initiative fatigue

A common theme across the whole SHARP programme was that communities had grown used to being the subject of research or regeneration activities that ultimately made little difference, except perhaps to confirm the stigmatising label of deprivation. Several of the projects were sited in areas that had been heavily researched in the past, often on the 'parachute model': researchers dropped in from outside, gathered their data and disappeared, with no long-term change resulting for the community. This had led to a high degree of scepticism among local residents that acted as an immense barrier, at least in the beginning, to successful engagement between projects and communities.

Triangle: research fatigue in Merthyr

In the Merthyr site that was one point of the Triangle, local residents had seen many research and development projects come to their area since the late 1960s, but little real improvement in living conditions. They had become cynical, which made it harder to engage them in new initiatives, as they felt that the time and effort they contributed would be wasted. Project field notes recorded the views of local residents:

"We've had six years of consultation and no benefit."

"Well, what's happened to all the other reports that have been fed back?"

People were aware that money was being spent on the area, but they did not see where it was going – except to the benefit of workers from outside who would leave the area at the end of the project. Decades of these experiences of disappointment had generated outright hostility and a feeling that more research was not what was needed, and in the early months of the project members of the project team experienced this directly. They reported encountering 'deep-rooted fatigue and alienation' (O'Neill and Williams, 2004, p 43). In some cases, this led to hostility, with residents expressing the view that money should be spent on improvements to the estate, not on consultation.

While some projects reported a sense of hostility to research from sections of their communities, this was not universal; there seemed to be little objection to the research activities in Right 2 Respect and BeWEHL. Community rejections of research are underreported in the literature: negative views may be unknown to senior academic practitioners, as fieldwork is normally the responsibility of research assistants (Boutilier et al, 1997). At local level, therefore, conventional research may have a 'bad press' and the potential for action has, beyond any doubt, been the main stimulus for the broader community involvement achieved by these projects.

In Pembrokeshire participants tended to perceive research as a high-status activity, enhanced through its links in this programme with the national government of Wales, but did express a certain fatigue with development initiatives and projects with short-term funding. The Monkton group lacked confidence about what the group could achieve. Members felt that vocal pessimists could drag it down. The community had seen initiatives, project workers and funding streams come and go, with little result on the ground. An action plan had been prepared in 2000, yet the same sorts of issues emerged during the SHARP interviews. The situation was succinctly described by one of the action researchers in Pembrokeshire:

> They [that is, communities/community groups] get thrown the most difficult circumstances to work with. People go and see them with all these expectations, and all these grants

come out, and this or that scheme is here, and out comes someone to work with them for a couple of years. And then they disappear. And then, 'ooh, there's this new funding stream'. And these communities don't know whether they're coming or going. (Carlisle et al, 2004, p 34)

Reciprocity

While those involved in running the various SHARP projects had engagement high on their agendas, the people living in the communities where the projects were working may have felt very differently. People may reject engagement for perfectly valid reasons, the strongest of which is simply because they cannot see any potential benefit from taking part. Community members have limited reserves of time and energy; in order to engage them, the SHARP projects had to find ways of conveying that that time and energy would be well spent on the project.

The Triangle project (see box below) tackled this at a very practical level. Other projects also emphasised the social aspects of research and action events. Barefoot put great emphasis on providing free lunch, as well as offering the chance for long-term personal development and ultimately the prospect of employment.

Triangle: leaves and light bulbs

The Triangle project tried to encourage people to become engaged in the process by making the whole process more reciprocal – integrating the research and activity elements of the action research process into what they called 'social event methodology'. This was a way of giving people something back, rather than just taking away information from them. What they got back was in some cases an immediate benefit – for example, low-energy kettles and light bulbs supplied by the local electricity company were handed out at a consultation event. It proved a very successful means of drawing over 300 people in, some queuing for over an hour before the event. They received not just electrical equipment, but also information about local services, and were invited to take part in a 'research tree' exercise. People wrote on leaf shaped papers what they thought were the best and the worst thing about living in the neighbourhood, and what one thing would most improve it, then stuck the papers to a tree. This approach ensured that people got back immediate feedback on the research process – not thick or rich data perhaps, but there, in front of people's eyes.

Community members know that they are working in a situation of inequality. In the Pembrokeshire SHARP project, community members commented on the contrast between the financial resources held by the project and the fact that they 'got nothing'. As in Holway, money was made available by the Pembrokeshire project as a 'community chest' for local groups to access, but there was no direct reward for individuals taking part in the engagement process, except for the small number who received a fee for carrying out interviews.

Leadership and 'gatekeepers' in the communities

Not all members of a community play equal roles in the processes of engagement. In any community, certain members may take on the role of speaking on behalf of others, sometimes with the overt consent of their peers, sometimes without. The various projects discovered that the role of community leaders may be a complex one, with authority assumed or granted in many different ways. Community leaders may take on the role of gatekeepers, with the ability either to facilitate or to block engagement between project workers and the community. In both Pembrokeshire and Triangle, for example, researchers discovered that a community may contain one powerful individual – unelected, unofficial – whose tacit blessing is required before other community members are willing to participate in the project. One of the action researchers in Pembrokeshire described his experience of trying to initiate engagement in the rural area:

> "One of the very interesting things that happened when I came into this community to try and get this project going, get this process started, was it was very obvious there was one individual in the village that was what I would term the 'gatekeeper'. And that person had a huge amount of respect from others in the community, and it didn't really matter who I spoke to in the community, they wanted me to speak to this one individual and they wanted to see what the outcome of that was. So it was very difficult to get things moving and get things going forward without having the full engagement of the gatekeeper. Which finally when that happened the project, it just flew." (Welsh Assembly Government, 2006)

The Barefoot project confronted a particularly complex set of gatekeepers. The project aimed to set up a Bangladeshi Reference Group with which the project could liaise and that would be representative of the whole community. However, there were already a number of groups operating within the Bangladeshi community in Cardiff. The conflicts and differences in opinion between these groups made it harder for the community to come together and to voice their common concerns collectively. Traditionally, certain sections of the community, such as women and young people, had not been involved or represented by these groups. Outside organisations and service providers looking to access the Bangladeshi community often approach these groups as a way into the community. This approach has often led to the information being left in the hands of the 'gatekeepers' with little or no access to the grass-roots level.

Measuring engagement and assessing its impact

The process of engagement may initially be viewed as an end in itself, but ultimately it has to be measured by the success achieved in bridging the differences and making connections between the various parties to the engagement. Engagement is seen as an essential part of the action research process, but it is worth asking whether it is the case that 'the more engagement the better' and whether there is a threshold level of engagement that is required for a project to be successful.

Engagement in the context of the SHARP programme can be considered in relation to Arnstein's (1969) 'ladder of participation' model, which considers the relationship between community members and organisations. In the 'ladder' model, each rung from the bottom to the top represents an increasing level of participation of members of the public in the design and running of services or interventions; it was introduced by Arnstein in her work looking at the relationship between citizens and planners, but the ideas are transferable to any public service activity. A simplified version of Arnstein's ladder is presented in the box opposite.

The ladder of participation

Model 'A' has the greatest degree of participation by community members, and 'F' the least.

A Users have control: users determine priorities, policies and strategies of the service. Users may recruit their own staff who are responsible to the users.

B Involvement in planning: involvement within a management committee or commissioning group in partnership with professionals. Individuals receive the care they want, rather than a 'prescription.'

C Part of the consultation process, with the ability to change agendas: open, well-publicised, wide-ranging consultation where ideas and opinions are listened to and acted on. Consultation is a continuous process, and users receive feedback.

D 'Tokenistic' consultation: opinions are canvassed on a small scale, similar to market research. Usually a one-way process with little or no feedback to users, and professional views are prioritised. Individuals may be persuaded to receive a certain type of service.

E Receipt of information: communication is a one-way process with users being informed of decisions being taken elsewhere.

F No involvement: services are offered on a 'take it or leave it' basis.

Source: adapted from Arnstein (1969) and Health Advisory Service (1997)

Arnstein's ladder presents a static or 'snapshot' view of the relationship between communities and organisations, glossing over the dynamic nature of the processes of engagement. However, it is useful because it throws into relief two issues at the heart of engagement, namely *power* and *control*. Moving from the bottom to the top of the ladder reflects a transfer of power from the organisation to the service user or citizen. Citizens involved in processes higher up the ladder gain power and control as an outcome of the involvement.

Although Arnstein argued powerfully that involvement should be taking place on the highest rungs of the ladder, she acknowledged that even there the outcomes may not be a pure or entirely effective form of citizen control. Community organisations taking over control can develop their own bureaucracies and internal politics and end up replicating the organisations they have replaced. The 'ladder of involvement' shows how shifts in the balance of power and control are – or should be – one of the intended outcomes of the engagement process. In SHARP, engagement has been an integral part of the action research process, a means to the end of bringing about change in communities' health and circumstances. This impact is summed up in the final project report on HYPP:

> The progress made by HYPP has been a testimony to the energy, enthusiasm and creativity of the children, who when given a platform and forum, have been able to articulate and develop ways of meeting their own needs and requirements. The overwhelming lesson to be drawn is that children themselves are a key resource when examining and promoting health-enhancing behaviour. (Goodwin and Armstrong-Esther, 2005, p 21)

In addition, engagement has shown its value as a process in its own right, contributing to increased confidence and the building of social capital (to be discussed in more detail in Chapter Eight). The overarching evaluation team described the valuable role of engagement in the Barefoot project, where both workers and stakeholders believed that the greatest impact of the project has been its:

> success in working collaboratively with people of all ages from particular groups, who have rarely been successfully engaged by other means or services. This inclusive but indirect approach to community health improvement has taken several years to build, pointing to the real difficulties of expecting short-term change from action research with marginalised social groups. Equally important, these new networks remain fragile relationships in need of nurturing. (Carlisle et al, 2005, p 67)

A third way in which the processes of engagement that took place through SHARP have, in many cases, made a difference is through their lasting impact on the structures of engagement that allow interaction between communities and public sector organisations of all types. In HYPP, children of all ages, and from different social, cultural and linguistic communities, came together to establish and run a youth council, Dyfodol Llanwyrtyd Future, and were invited to address town council meetings in order to express their requirements concerning local services and activities. They have also managed to connect themselves to 'influential others', locally, regionally and even nationally – in addition to their invitations to Cardiff Bay and Westminster, a member of Dyfodol now sits on the council of Funky Dragon, the Welsh Assembly's consultation group for young people across Wales.

This outcome is similar to that achieved by the Women in Action group facilitated by both the Triangle and Barefoot projects. The group has now succeeded in positioning itself in a role that has high-profile and meaningful connection with the local authority, the Local Public Health Team of the National Public Health Service and all levels of the National Assembly for Wales. Evidence of this was the list of those who attended a seminar in which Women in Action set out its background, achievements and future aspirations.

Conclusion

The various SHARP projects revealed the complexities of the processes of engagement between projects and communities. Their experiences highlighted the ways in which engagement is integral to action research. They showed that engagement with a community can only ever be partial and, to some degree, partisan, and that a degree of pragmatism must shape the projects' ambitions for engagement. They demonstrated the ways in which 'depth' of engagement – intensively, with a small number of people – can be a more realistic and effective ideal than 'breadth' of engagement with a larger number of people, but at a more superficial level.

Engagement may need to be managed carefully, and expectations limited. Working on community engagement may entail dealing with and resolving conflicting values and priorities. There may be differences of priorities held by different members within a community. There may be values held by some community members that are at odds with the values of the service planners, providers or funders. Engagement does not automatically lead to the outcomes people hope for. It can raise hopes that, if they are not met, can lead to disillusionment. The SHARP projects demonstrated that engagement, and community members' expectations of it, had to be carefully managed. In the Holway project, for example, the single most important issue identified by residents at the start of the project was the state of pre-cast concrete houses on the estate. Only at the end of the project – four years down the line – was the council beginning to address this.

Three of the projects (Triangle, Barefoot, Pembrokeshire) took a very particular approach to tackling engagement, by choosing to recruit local community researchers to act as links between the communities, the projects and the respective organisations within which each project was based. The next chapter goes on to discuss these workers, and their roles as key players making links between projects and communities and also negotiating with gatekeepers in the communities.

References

Arnstein, S. (1969) 'A ladder of citizen participation in the USA', *Journal of the American Institute of Planners*, vol 35, no 4, pp 216-24.

Barnes, M., Newman, J. and Sullivan, H. (2007) *Power, Participation and Political Renewal*, Bristol: The Policy Press.

Carlisle, S., Cropper, S., Beech, R. and Little, R. (2004, unpublished) 'SHARP Overarching Evaluation Team Phase 2 Report', Keele: Keele University.

Carlisle, S., Cropper, S., Beech, R. and Little, R. (2005) *Investing in Sustainable Health Action Research in Wales: Final Report on Phases 1 & 2 of the Sustainable Health Action Research Programme*, Cardiff: WAG.

Cohen, A.P. (1985) *The Symbolic Construction of Community*, London: Routledge and Kegan Paul.

Emmel, N. (2004) *Toward Community Involvement: Strategies for Health and Social Care Providers – Guide 2, The Complexity of Communities and Lessons for Community Involvement*, Leeds: Nuffield Institute for Health.

Emmel, N. and Conn, C. (2004) *Towards Community Involvement: Strategies for Health and Social Care Providers – Guide 1, Identifying the Goals and Objectives of Community Involvement*, Leeds: Nuffield Institute for Health.

Goodwin, M. and Armstrong-Esther, D. (2005) *SHARP Phase 2 Report – Health of Young People in Powys*, http://new.wales.gov.uk/docrepos/40382/cmo/reports/2006/hypp-report?lang=en (accessed 27 July 2007).

Health Advisory Service (1997) *Voices in Partnership*, London: The Stationery Office.

Jewkes, R. and Murcott, A. (1996) 'Meanings of community', *Social Science and Medicine*, vol 43, no 4, pp 555-63.

ODPM (Office of the Deputy Prime Minister) (2003) *Searching for Solid Foundations: Community Involvement and Urban Policy*, London: ODPM.

O'Neill, M. and Williams, G. (2004) 'Developing community and agency engagement in an action research study', *Critical Public Health*, vol 14, pp 37-48.

Popay, J., Thomas, C., Williams, G., Bennett, S., Gatrell, A. and Bostock, L. (2003) 'A proper place to live: health inequalities, agency and the normative dimensions of space', *Social Science and Medicine*, vol 57, pp 55-69.

Rogers, B. and Robinson, E. (2004) *The Benefits of Community Education: A Review of the Evidence*, London: Civil Renewal Unit, Home Office.

Smyth, J. (2001) *Social Capital and Community Involvement*, Paper for Audit Commission seminar held on 4 December, ww2.audit-commission.gov.uk/pis/doc/pi_q/socialcapital.doc (accessed on 27 July 2007)

Welsh Assembly Government (2006) 'SHARP: working together to improve our lives', DVD Dart Film and Video, Cardiff: Welsh Assembly Government.

Wilmott, P. and Thomas, D. (1984) *Community in Social Policy*, London: Policy Studies Institute.

SIX

The role of the community-based action researcher

Martin O'Neill

Introduction

The value and importance of involving communities in the development and delivery of policies that affect them is increasingly being recognised, and this is reflected in policy directives (Welsh Office, 1998; DH, 2001). Throughout the development of the Sustainable Health Action Research Programme (SHARP), there was an emphasis on involving communities substantially and directly in an action research process aimed at tackling the health and wellbeing issues they faced. In Chapter Five, Bronwen Bermingham and Alison Porter set out some of SHARP's learning about working with communities. This chapter focuses on one particular way in which projects sought to engage communities in the action research process and discusses the role and experiences of community-based action researchers (CBARs).

The classic model of action research advocates that participants engage in an ongoing iterative, cyclical or 'helical' process of action and reflection/evaluation that then informs practice (Kemmis and McTaggart, 2000). In theory, such an approach to participatory research should be characterised by openness to change and acceptance of an unpredictability of outcomes. The approach is also generally taken to imply the active participation of research 'subjects' in decisions about research questions, design and conduct (Cornwall and Jewkes, 1995; Boutilier et al, 1997; Dick, 1999; Stoecker, 2003); in these, 'indigenous proficiencies' are valued (Ansari et al, 2002). Yet, as much of the literature on participatory forms of research with communities makes clear, primary responsibility tends to remain within the academic and/or professional community (Lindsey and McGuiness, 1998; Cheadle et al, 2002; Krieger et al, 2002; Schultz et al, 2002; Mumford et al, 2003; Savan, 2004). Within much of the literature in the field, there appears to be little reference to the role of the lay researcher other than as a data collector, as a 'research associate', or, when academic researchers work with other language communities, as an 'interpreter' (Jones and Allebone, 1999).

Although there were a number of variations on the model of action developed within SHARP, this chapter draws on the experience of three of the projects – Barefoot, Triangle and Pembrokeshire – that either employed, or engaged on a voluntary basis, members of communities who were then intimately involved in developing action research within their community.

The CBAR model was felt to be particularly appropriate for the types of setting in which the SHARP projects were based – communities that had been a concern to public agencies for some time, for reasons of deprivation or social and economic exclusion, poor access to services, or a lack of cohesion – because it offered, potentially, a way of addressing a growing unwillingness to participate in social research (Cook, 2004). In general, more collaborative research strategies, such as action research, may, if employed effectively, help to counter this escalation of research fatigue. Action research, in particular, offers a more direct exchange than 'extractive research', in that it seeks to address not only the questions of the researcher but also to contribute to pressing issues faced by those who are collaborating in the research enterprise. But the first task is to connect with the community and to establish a relationship of collaboration.

The CBARs had three important characteristics:

- they combined, in one person's responsibilities, the action and research functions of the project, at least to some degree;
- they 'belonged' to the community;
- they were, at least at the start of each appointment, seen as 'lay' rather than professional researchers.

As the rest of this chapter will argue, none of these characteristics is straightforward. Combining the action and research roles proved challenging, and confusing, with priorities unclear to the CBARs. The notion of 'belonging' to a community raised questions about representativeness, and also presented difficult challenges to the researchers around mixed loyalties and the risk of betrayal. The fact that the CBARs were 'lay' had implications not just for skills training, but also meant that they had a difficult task of straddling and trying to reconcile two very different cultural spheres, academia and the community, and the expectations that each implicitly, or indeed explicitly, held.

As the pen sketches of the SHARP projects in Chapter Three indicated, the 'Barefoot' Health Workers project was based in an area of Cardiff with a diverse cultural mix, a large percentage of the population being from black and minority ethnic (BME) groups. The minority ethnic groups with which the project chose to work were the Bangladeshi, Somali and Yemeni communities, most of whose members are Muslim. The project was named after the community researchers/health advisers to reflect their centrality to the project, although the cultural and religious connotations of going barefoot to the communities involved had not initially been understood; had they been understood, another name would have surely been sought. For each community, an individual with relevant experience, commitment and the resourcefulness to undertake community health development and research activity was recruited; although one woman with health research experience was recruited, the majority of community researchers had experience of community leadership. In total, during the lifetime of the project, five different SHARP action researchers were involved in the project, as two of the initial recruits left the project. Triangle took a similar approach, recruiting one CBAR from (and for) each of the three communities in the project; in contrast with the Barefoot project, all three workers, employed by Cardiff University but based in their respective communities, stayed for the duration of the project and this gave both continuity and sustained momentum to Triangle's work in the three communities.

The approach in the SHARP Pembrokeshire project was somewhat different; the CBARs had a more limited role, recruited to carry out interviews and analyse the data arising, but with no expectation that they would catalyse and support action in their communities. The 14 researchers were not employed, but were paid a fixed fee per interview completed or attempted. Many of them stayed on with the project on a voluntary basis after the end of the interviewing phase.

Expectations and challenges

The development of a CBAR model within SHARP was based on the rationale that, although local people may not have formal research skills or qualifications, good local knowledge, community roots, contacts and connections, motivation to work for the community's benefit, and other 'indigenous proficiencies' were much more important. In Salford and Nottinghamshire, the Social Action Research Project (SARP) had used a similar approach and had worked with local projects to explore the links between health, wellbeing and social capital. The research that SARP conducted highlighted the importance of engaging already established networks and groups and working with them in order to evaluate their activity and develop further action (Boeck and Fleming, 2002). The main assumptions associated with the CBAR role within the overall action research process can be categorised as falling under three main headings:

- **Networks:** They would be able to draw on forms of knowledge and social networks/relationships not accessible to 'outsider' researchers. Because of this, they would be well placed to define what was needed and likely to work in each community and to encourage participation by others in the community in action.
- **Skills:** During the course of project implementation, lay researchers would develop practical skills in community development, action research and evaluative techniques, and would be able to gather information to help demonstrate and assess the effectiveness of actions and adjust these as needed.
- **Legacy:** Their skills and networks would be left with the individuals and community after the programme ended, as a beneficial, longer-term legacy.

Although the CBARs brought a lot of local knowledge to the projects, they still found that because they were taking on a new role within their communities, it was necessary to devote the early stages simply to meeting and listening to local people. The CBARs were in a role that was new to them and so they found that they heard (listened to) and understood the most pressing wellbeing issues, the cultural and social norms that influenced these views and people's responses to them in a different way. In their new role, they also had to explain to members of the local community how their role was different from what they may have been doing before – where, for example, they had been volunteers for services within their communities.

Where the projects did not give CBARs an early data collection task, or one that took them to the doors of people in their community, the development of relationships and a recognised presence took a period of time. The slow and cautious start was occasionally frustrating for some of those involved who felt that agency expectations in relation to outputs and outcomes did not value the importance of building relationships. In retrospect, however, the work to build understanding of the role and the project was critical to ensuring that when the first tentative actions were encouraged, they resonated with local people.

CBARs spent significant time and effort working out how to integrate and reintegrate themselves into various community groupings and how to develop and coordinate their ongoing activities in a practical way. They also had to account for their time to management groups that could not fully grasp the situation they were trying to operate in. These situations proved both stressful and isolating for the CBARs. Fostering social cohesion and a sense of group ownership among diverse social groups required skill and sensitivity from the CBARs. They developed a keen intuitive understanding of the support needs of individuals as well as the group as a whole. To do this, it was useful that they had a close identity with the group that might involve taking responsibility for supporting activities, securing resources and so on, and that would also mean that they routinely participated in activities and events. They found that the relationships they formed and the insights they gained from spending time with the various community members guided them through the subtle processes of group formation and dynamics.

Developing innovative action research, particularly where it is highly participatory, poses considerable personal and institutional challenges for those involved. Although action research of this kind is in many ways very different from conventional research, there are also skills and competences that need to be acquired and demonstrated to other people participating in the research, if it is to be taken seriously. The CBARs needed to become adept at cooperation, open communication, intellectual rigour and personal persistence. Despite the very marked differences that existed between the communities that were involved in the SHARP programme, the participatory approaches across the projects functioned and developed in very similar ways in many situations. Three key issues emerged from the action research process that were particularly difficult to manage:

- balancing insider/outsider identities and roles;
- negotiating and managing power differentials;
- action versus research.

While certain aspects of these are features of any social research process, there are tensions and ambiguities in setting up a research process that is explicitly community-driven, reciprocal and participative, which create particular ambiguities and tensions for the research role.

Insider/outsider identities and roles

Unlike most academic researchers, CBARs were not strangers within the community. As the example below from Pembrokeshire suggests, the 'insider' status of CBARs proved in some cases to be even more significant than those who designed the projects bargained for:

Pembrokeshire SHARP: in or out of your own area

Pembrokeshire project researchers were recruited from what were identified as two different communities. Once they started interviewing, however, they swapped, so that all the researchers were interviewing outside their own neighbourhood. This was meant to preserve anonymity, and save any potential embarrassment during the interviews. However, it soon became clear that there were problems with this approach. Some of these were practical, with those interviewers without cars finding the arrangements particularly time-consuming and awkward. More significantly, researchers reported that working outside their own neighbourhood seemed to be putting a block on engaging with people. Community members seemed 'wary of strangers' and 'didn't want to get involved'. At the request of the community researchers, the areas were swapped back, so people were interviewing in their own neighbourhoods. One researcher recounted:

> "When I did my first interview in [her home community] I realised that this is what I had thought the job would actually be like. It was much easier, and the people either knew my children or me, and were much more willing to talk (though they did need some extra persuading). I really felt that I was doing something good for the community and tried to convey this to the interviewees."

Although by definition the people who took on the role of CBAR were resident in the area, or otherwise defined as community members, by taking the role into practice they were making themselves different from others in the community: for example, recording and reflecting on what has been said and done is not something that community members do as a matter of course. This in itself produced feelings of doubt and uncertainty. For example, CBARs reported that when they started writing and talking about their experiences and taking these descriptions outside their communities they were uneasy, even though it was part of their job description. They felt that they were being traitors to their own communities. Even recognising this was discomforting: the researchers were not accustomed to writing about and sharing such personal feelings, particularly with someone who lived outside their community who was their line manager.

The CBARs found that managing this insider/outsider identity was something that had to be continually negotiated and renegotiated. At times, even those who, on the face of it, had strong local credentials began to get the message that more established community members resented their efforts. For example, they were defined as 'newcomers' who lacked the social and political legitimacy of those who had been born and lived their whole lives in the locality. They were therefore not regarded as having the understanding, right or authority to change 'the way things have always been done'. For others, the challenge came from established community leaders, who wanted to approve or veto activities and consultations CBARs had organised. Although various strategies were used to overcome such 'political' barriers, as Chapter Five noted, this proved to be something that needed constant management as the CBAR moved through and between the different social spheres in which they needed to operate.

The development of a CBAR is not a case simply of training local people in research methods and providing continuing supervision, while insider status and knowledge help in maintaining standards of research. This does not reflect the complex criteria that define the individual and communal construction of the insider. Within the literature on participatory approaches to community development there appears to be an assumption that researchers will encounter consensus within the community. But, as Chapter Five argued, communities are not homogeneous. They are characterised by gender, ethnic, religious, social and spatial divisions. A key skill that the CBARs needed to develop was the ability to manage the social divisions that existed and work around them. The alliances and antagonisms that demarcated these divisions could be very deep and have long histories and could run along tensions based on spatial or ethnic groups or on long-standing family and personal differences or animosities.

CBARs were very aware of community boundaries and membership criteria and the impact of their role on the way they were judged. Of their communities, for example, they noted that 'different BME [black and minority ethnic] communities don't stick together', and remarked on differences in generations, differences due to dialect and geographical region of origin, and differences in rugby club affiliation. Of their relationship with their communities, CBARs had been 'selected' not only by the employing project, but also, well into the project, by their communities on the basis of community credentials rather than qualifications: 'they would ask who is that person's father, what does he do'.

It is unsurprising that 'managing the self' in such situations leads to feelings of uncertainty, because it is making conscious and explicit the routine encounters of daily life. Interactions become defined both as part of a job of work and as friendship or neighbourliness: where agencies demand 'professionalism', the expectations in the community may rest solely on previous roles and relationships.

Moreover, in these long-term, community-based projects, the CBARs were intensely involved with individuals and groups, privy to the details of the lives of people with whom they may have a variety of bases on which they relate. Distinguishing legitimate data from personal confidences was difficult. Due to this attenuation of the boundaries between researcher and researched, both on a personal and project level, there was often no clear distinction of roles and no clear guidelines of how to manage the tensions that it generated. CBARs also reported that their role seemed to lead them to develop false intimacy with others in the community, and they had concerns about the ramifications this might have for continuing to live in the community, particularly when researching extremely sensitive subject areas. This issue becomes further complicated when put into a broader cultural context of knowing when and where to expose particular facets of one's self within particular social situations. The experiences of those involved in the SHARP projects suggests that managing competing and constantly shifting insider/outsider identities and perspectives is a key challenge for those who seek to develop the CBAR approach.

Negotiating and managing power differentials

At community level, managing power dynamics was a prime concern for the CBARs. For example, while all the CBARs possessed local knowledge and social contacts, none was an established community leader. They had to develop support networks and partnership structures within their community. One of the researchers from the Barefoot project recounted how important it was to get community leaders on board: "If a project or activity has the support of the imams and senior men, it will work. If not, it's doomed to failure".

In many ways, the CBARs had to learn to steer a difficult course between different power structures – many deeply institutionalised, including those around religion, ethnic identity and gender – all of which were complex. One CBAR working in a minority ethnic community commented that: "All groups within the community are led by men. I really thought I would struggle," but added: "There are internal tensions within the community – political allegiance, religious, etc. I think it's easier for women. There's always more of a threat with a man – more respect.... I think if a man was doing this job, the impact and activities would be different."

Some CBARs reported feeling that they were being used by those who were directing the research, whether in a university or a health service agency. There was a view that the provision of training was motivated more by instrumental concerns about collecting data than any genuine attempt to give power to people in the community. Occasionally CBARs recounted that they felt relationships within the projects were hierarchical, and they were being expected to report and reflect on their roles in a way in which other team members were not.

This situation is indicative of some of the inherent power differentials contained within action research. Although the professed aim of participatory action research is to 'empower' people and communities so they can participate as equals in the process, unsurprisingly, there are power differences that make such parity difficult to achieve, however well intentioned. In the more macro research environment of the real world, this is a complex position to attain as it inherently challenges the power dynamics in the traditional research model where an elite group – social scientists, health services researchers or health promotion professionals – exclusively or at least predominantly determine the form and process of research.

In some cases, CBARs found themselves struggling with the fears of academic partners that they were 'going native' – identifying too strongly with the values and aims of the researched. The term has an 'othering' connotation that is contrary to the ethos of a participatory approach that seeks to establish a consensus, based on equality of status, where the aims of the researchers and the researched coalesce. Besides, the CBARs, by definition, started out as 'natives'; the tension around the concept reveals as much about partners' assumptions as it does about the role and activities of the CBARs.

As an example of the sometimes competing motivations that emerge in such a collaborative research endeavour, ultimately an academic's career and a university's funding is dependent on the number of publications they produce and research grants they attract. The production of academic outputs, however, is of little consequence to those outside the academic community; their desired outputs tend to be more immediate and material and aimed at addressing needs, as all the SHARP projects found. In addition, all the projects involved other agencies – Local Health Boards (the Welsh variant of England's Primary Care Trusts), the police, local authority housing or social services departments – and partnerships such as Local Health Alliances (a Welsh organisational mechanism to bring local stakeholders together) that all have agendas they wish to satisfy via the research process. Research commissioners or healthcare agencies, for instance, require research reports produced in language that may well mean very little to others who have participated in their production.

In addition, the location of the project budget and who has control over it will understandably have implications for the overall power dynamic of the action research process. Our experiences have taught us that it is probably impossible to attain a situation where all these multiple agendas can be replaced by one participatory schema, but adopting a shared approach to managing these different agendas and the inherent tensions that these produce can result in a mutually enlightening experience for all those concerned. Managing the perceived and real power differential between the research institutions and the community is of crucial importance, not only for the successful employment of action research methodology, but also for the social and personal wellbeing of the CBARs. The action research experience is one of learning both for participants and for researchers, and as such if executed effectively, should lead to joint action and learning. Accepting uncertainty is an important and vital part of developing participative techniques, as control does not rest with one group or individual.

Action versus research

Managing the competing demands for action versus research was a strategic issue for the whole SHARP initiative, but it was also very evident as a dilemma faced by individual CBARs, since community expectations of concrete action were high. However, successfully delivering that action was often beyond what the CBARs could achieve by themselves. Sometimes the lack of linkage between research and action could have implications for the credibility of CBARs within their community and led to personal feelings of frustration:

> "It's a tension that runs through the whole thing, because in theory we are researchers, we're not development workers. And there is no development role in this project. But if there's nobody there doing the development role, there's

nothing there to evaluate." (Community researcher, Triangle project)

The CBARs probably felt the inherent tension between the 'action' and the 'research' components of the process particularly acutely because they operated at the cutting edge of the competing demands that caused the split loyalties to their communities and to the research institutions that employed or engaged them. Failing to deliver effective action proved to be the biggest obstacle to maintaining participation at all levels. This demand for action at community level meant that it was difficult for the CBAR to engage in the reflection and evaluation aspect of the action research process. However, from experience we found that if meaningful, effective, sustainable action was to be developed, it was crucial for evaluation of the process to be integrated into the project from the start.

Community researchers spoke of an initial period of profound uncertainty about the meaning and character of action research and the ways in which it should be practised. Was community-based action research about systematic data gathering followed by action, or a cycle of organising and action followed by reflection on that action? Was research an ongoing activity, or episodic and sporadic, based on action on particular issues? What were CBARs supposed to evaluate and in what terms? Were they supposed to evaluate specific activities for their contribution to community health, or the process of identifying priorities and mobilising for action? The sheer difficulty of holding 'action' and 'research' together coherently was an anxiety also experienced by project leaders, including academics who could not provide the clarity of guidance the CBARs were looking for. Many of the CBARs initially expressed negative views about the research element of action research, despite support and encouragement from project management. These views changed over time, as they came to appreciate what action research could add to community health development work:

> "When I first started, I thought it should all be community development. The community should benefit, not the academics. But I can see that the skills they've taught me – reflecting, recording, consulting as second nature – that produces better community development. I couldn't see the relevance of it at first. Now, two years later, I can. Action research is just common sense, really – thinking about how you do a job properly – but the difference is that we write about it. It forces you to be more organised in your

> reflecting. You're producing something that you're feeding back to people – that's the usefulness of it." (Community researcher, Triangle project)

Some CBARs recounted that they had little idea how to link or coordinate efforts and felt that they were provided with inadequate support, guidance or supervision. They reported feeling 'torn' and 'inadequate', as they were unsure that they were doing the 'right thing'. This uncertainty and 'messiness' of the reality encountered was something that needed to be managed and accepted as part of the process. The classical model of participatory action research theorises it as an ongoing cyclical phased process consisting of research, reflection and action. In reality, this rarely happened in a neatly structured process and this precipitated feelings of uncertainty for the CBARs. Many of the SHARP projects and activities incorporated all stages of the action research cycle (in some cases several turns of the cycle) and this sometimes made people feel that things were not happening or that the process was out of control. Nonetheless, particularly in retrospect, the various stages could be observed; more importantly, however, the sustainability and success of the actions developed were clearly influenced by the action approach and process.

Developing into the role of CBAR

Identifying and employing individuals who were insiders was rarely straightforward. Traditional advertising failed to attract suitable applicants for the posts – those that tended to apply had research qualifications and backgrounds, and were too 'outside' the rest of the community. Although, on occasion, suitable candidates from the community were identified by the project team, they needed to be persuaded to apply for the post. The Triangle project, for instance, found that when it attempted to recruit a CBAR – under the job title 'Local Sustainable Health Coordinator' – through an advert in the local press, it didn't produce any applicants from the community they were seeking to work in. It seemed that potential applicants were put off by the job title, and by the fact that a university some miles away from where they lived was to be the employer. Additionally, the standard application form for a research assistant asked about people's formal qualifications and what degree they had. These were implicit personal and institutional barriers that needed to be overcome and continually resolved in order to engage with 'insiders'. Similarly, in Pembrokeshire, potential CBARs appeared to feel inhibited about applying, as one of them reported:

"My young son brought me home a leaflet from school. When I read it, it said they were looking for community researchers in our local community. It sounded like a challenge so I phoned for an application form, never thought I stood a chance. I had no qualifications, GCSEs or O levels, I work in our local hospital as a domestic and do some healthcare work on my days off, but I thought why not try anyway, the application form was straightforward and I told them a bit about myself. The day of the interview I was nervous but was put at ease, three people interviewed me and each in turn asked me some questions. The whole thing lasted about 30 minutes and they said I would hear soon. Not for one moment did I think I would get the job, I am just your ordinary every day person I surely won't get the job. So I was amazed when the letter came and they said I got the job." (Community researcher, Pembrokeshire project)

In a small number of cases, initial appointments left after a short time in the post, for a number of reasons. Those who settled into the role had to be acceptable not only to the community but also to other project partners. These challenges of recruiting and retaining CBARs affected the progress, momentum and continuity in the research process.

Community-based action research requires a number of very different skills. While this was understood by those who were recruited to the role of CBAR, direct experience of, and skills in, research, especially in participative methods of working, were generally low at the outset. Project leaders and CBARs were unsure what sort of training would be most appropriate to the role they were developing. It was found that university-based training in either action research or community development was less valuable than a general, practical introduction to participatory data collection and analysis. Despite the relative inexperience in participative techniques of most of the CBARs, this initial training was quickly built on, adapted and augmented. In Pembrokeshire, CBARs both qualified with an Open College Network Level 2 Certificate and wrote their own guide to community research. In Barefoot and Triangle, they quickly began to develop innovative and context-specific techniques for data collection and implementing the action research approach in general based on their local knowledge, with little need for further input from the 'professional' researchers.

Despite receiving some training, the process of learning to do action research seems, for community researchers, to be both daunting and, potentially, damaging to self-esteem:

"That confusion you get with action research – you don't know what the hell you're doing. And there's the self-doubts…. Am I up to the job? Am I doing it right?" (Community researcher, Triangle project)

The CBARs reported that they had gained confidence in their personal ability and skills: "I've learnt a skill and [made] friends at the same time….When we had our certificates, I never felt so important in my life". They also recognised that the skills they already possessed had been enhanced and developed through their work: these included various skills related to working in the community through listening, communication, mentoring and learning to suspend judgement on other people's views and behaviour.

CBARs also reported that they felt that their work had enabled them to improve their employment prospects (a number remain employed on community-based projects), or to continue with participation in learning (for example, two enrolled for counselling courses), while others became more involved in voluntary and community activities.

Conclusion

Those SHARP projects that used the CBAR model found that it worked: the CBARs gave projects an entrée into communities, and brought a very different perspective from that which would have been provided by 'traditional' researchers. From the point of view of the individuals involved, the role of CBAR offered opportunities for personal and career development. But the impact of the CBAR role on both projects and individuals was complex. There are social risks and ethical issues to be considered as well as functional considerations.

The CBAR model puts a heavy expectation on the researchers, to embody two of the fundamental principles of action research – integrating the action and research functions, and putting community members at the centre of the process. Simply being from a community does not imply that someone has access to or understanding of the whole community. Taking on a CBAR role could change the way in which people were perceived by their neighbours, as well as how they saw themselves. CBARs came up against doubts, fear of betrayal and confusion (their own and project partners') with their role. Some also found difficulties with placing limits, in terms of availability and function, on their role as CBARs, while at the same time maintaining their role as community member, 24 hours a day, seven days a week and with no job description.

While employing CBARs did not automatically give the researchers access to all areas of the community in an easy and unproblematic way, the knowledge and expertise the local researchers brought to the process gave other members of the team early insight into the indigenous power structures at play within the communities and how best to work around them to deliver effective action. In addition, as the CBARs developed various community initiatives, they were able to build on and maintain their position and standing within the community, while at the same time extending their networks into other groupings and agencies in order to ensure effective delivery of action. The CBARs were best placed to manage this delicate balance between consultation and action because their ears were close to the ground and they could best appreciate the contextual contingencies of the environment that they were working in.

The CBARs assumed an important role in their communities and filled an organisational void. Despite the challenges presented to us and to the community groups, most communities appear to have positively assessed their experiences in relation to the projects working in their localities, and can point to a number of significant achievements that resulted either directly or indirectly from the SHARP programme. The employment of CBARs was a significant step forward for those communities involved. In many instances, those who took the role of the CBAR position have gone to build on their work and become effective 'community champions'.

Towards the end of the projects, when the CBARs reviewed the activity they had been involved in and the people they had worked with, most were generally surprised at how much had been accomplished. It was, though, very difficult to determine whether the accomplishments in each community could be attributed directly (or even indirectly) to activities developed by CBARs. Interestingly, this did not seem to be a major concern for most of them. They seemed to see activity developed by the CBARs not so much as a defining moment but rather as part of a wider and more organic effort directed towards community change. Through the process, community members were able to define for themselves what they saw as the most significant problems affecting their communities, and then define what they understood as both appropriate and sustainable solutions. We strongly believe that the participatory approaches adopted were responsible for this. Yet the role of the CBAR is also not without its unique and hidden set of challenges. The transformative, democratic possibilities inherent in participatory approaches create contradictions and dilemmas that need to be 'worked' and managed.

References

Boeck, T. and Fleming, J. (2002) *Social Capital and the Nottingham Social Action Research Project*, Nottingham: Nottingham City Primary Care Trust.

Boutilier, M., Mason, R. and Rootman, I. (1997) 'Community action and reflective practice in health promotion research', *Health Promotion International*, vol 12, pp 69-78.

Cook, L. (2004) Discussion on the meeting on 'The 2001 Census and beyond', *Journal of the Royal Statistical Society: Series A (Statistics in Society)*, vol 167, no 2, pp 229-48.

Cornwall, A. and Jewkes, R. (1995) 'What is participatory research?', *Social Science & Medicine*, vol 41, pp 1667-76.

DH (Department of Health) (2001) *Tackling Health Inequalities: Consultation on a Plan for Delivery*, London: The Stationery Office.

Dick, B. (1999) 'What is action research?', www.scu.edu.au/schools/gcm/ar/whatisar.html

El Ansari, W., Phillips, C.J. and Zwi, A.B. (2002) 'Narrowing the gap between academic professional wisdom and community lay knowledge: perceptions from partnerships', *Public Health*, vol 116, pp 151-9.

Jones, L. and Allebone, B. (1999) 'Researching "hard-to-reach" groups: the crucial role of the research associate', *International Journal of Inclusive Education*, vol 3, no 4, pp 353-62.

Kemmis, S. and McTaggart, R. (2000) 'Participatory action research', in N. Denzin and Y. Lincoln (eds) *Handbook of Qualitative Research* (2nd edn), Thousand Oaks, CA: Sage Publications, pp 567-605.

Krieger, J., Allen, C., Cheadle, A., Ciske, S., Schier, J.K., Senturia, K. and Sullivan, M. (2002) 'Using community-based participatory research to address social determinants of health: lessons learned from Seattle Partners for Healthy Communities', *Health Education & Behavior*, vol 29, no 3, pp 361-82.

Lindsey, E. and McGuinness, L. (1998) 'Significant elements of community involvement in participatory action research: evidence from a community project', *Journal of Advanced Nursing*, vol 28, no 5, pp 1106-14.

Mumford, R. and Sanders, J. with Andrew, A. (2003) 'Community development – action research in community settings', *Social Work Education*, vol 22, pp 93-104.

Savan, B. (2004) 'Community–university partnerships: linking research and action for sustainable development', *Community Development Journal*, vol 39, no 4, pp 372-84.

Schulz, A., Krieger, J. and Galea, S. (2002) 'Addressing social determinants of health: community-based participatory approaches to research and practice', *Health Education & Behavior*, vol 29, no 3, pp 287-95.

Stoecker, R. (2003) 'Are academics irrelevant? Approaches and roles for scholars in community based participatory research', in M. Minkler and N. Wallerstein (eds) *Community-based Participatory Research for Health*, San Francisco, CA: Jossey Bass, pp 98-112.

Welsh Office (1998) *Better Health – Better Wales*, Cm 3922, Cardiff: The Stationery Office.

SEVEN

Evaluation, evidence and learning in community-based action research

Sandra Carlisle, Helen Snooks, Angela Evans and David Cohen

Introduction

Policy makers, professionals of all kinds and the general public now recognise a wide range of social factors as important determinants of health; if community health interventions can help to address such factors, they can play a valuable role in protecting and improving health and wellbeing (Shediac-Rizkallah and Bone, 1998). Publicly funded approaches that develop community capacity and connectedness may also promote stronger partnerships between communities and service providers, potentially leading to more appropriate forms of service provision. Yet, despite a high volume of research across the UK and elsewhere describing the problem of health inequalities, there is still comparatively little intervention research that helps to identify practical responses. There is also a growing expectation of 'evidence-based practice', which exerts great pressure to evaluate the effectiveness of community-level health interventions, although with regard to 'what works' at community level, there is a gap between the rhetoric of evidence-based policy and what happens on the ground, which is known to be far more complicated (Coote et al, 2004). There are thus questions about how such interventions should be evaluated and what constitutes 'evidence', especially when applied to novel approaches such as action research.

The SHARP initiative has focused on generating learning and evidence from community-based action research that will be of use for policy and practice to address health inequalities. This chapter argues that learning and evidence can take many forms in this type of intervention, so we need to cultivate a broader understanding of what works, for whom, and at what cost. The philosophy, assumptions and principles on which community-level research is based have implications for both methodology and methods, and therefore the evidence produced.

We begin by summarising some challenges in evaluating community-based initiatives to improve health and wellbeing. We then introduce the question of what constitutes evidence and learning in the community setting for action research provided through the Sustainable Health Action Research Programme (SHARP). We describe the different approaches to evaluation and evidence taken by participants in one project, and by the overarching evaluation team whose responsibility it was to draw comparative lessons from all seven. We explain the different purposes and principles underpinning these levels of evaluation, the forms of evaluation questions asked, and the links between these and methodological choices around design, process and conduct. Finally, we consider the opportunities and difficulties involved in transferring evidence from community-based action research to other contexts, for example for use by communities, policy makers, service providers and practitioners in service and policy development.

Evaluating community-level health interventions: mission impossible?

There is a well-known tendency for community health development programmes to be classified as failures (Rifkin, 1996; Zakus and Lysack, 1998). This may be because of misplaced assumptions about the nature of communities and unrealistic expectations around what community participation can achieve (Cohen, 1985; Jewkes and Murcott, 1998; Morgan, 2001). Such programmes are rarely designed to deliver a single intervention with one specific goal: they can be made up of a wide range of activities and projects, and draw on different fields and knowledge bases (such as health promotion, community development and urban regeneration) (Hills, 2004). In this context, the evaluation of such interventions is widely recognised as challenging (Robinson and Hill, 1995; Hepworth, 1997; Wimbush and Watson, 2000; Labonte, 2001; White, 2001).

'The community' can involve multiple stakeholders and shifting power relations, leading to complex sets of social processes. Community-based health initiatives can be as much about establishing an infrastructure (of community groups, partnerships between agencies, and new cross-cutting structures) as about the delivery of services to individuals (Hills, 2004). In this context, community development and capacity building can be viewed as an end in itself and a valid focus for evaluation. However, although community-based health interventions tend to focus on 'positive health' or 'health-as-wellbeing', they may use outcome measures or indicators of change, such as individual behaviour change, that do not reflect community priorities. There are also difficulties for evaluators in attributing change and in connecting cause with effect, as some outcomes may not be obvious for many years. Moreover, the time delay means that outcomes cannot be firmly linked to earlier interventions because of extraneous events that happen during the period.

Although the term 'evaluation' broadly refers to the process of determining the merit, worth or value of a programme and/or its products, three different types of purpose can be distinguished (Chelimsky, 1997):

- to provide accountability;
- to enable development (for example, providing evaluative help to strengthen institutions or programmes);
- to generate knowledge (for example, obtaining a deeper understanding of some specific area or policy).

A recent review of evaluations of community health initiatives suggests that many are carried out to inform local management (that is, an accountability purpose), rather than to produce broader and more generalisable knowledge (Hills, 2004). This 'local' purpose means that publication of findings, which contribute to the body of knowledge concerning what works in this field, is rare. The local approach may also entail problems with rigour: of design, data collection and reporting. There is the potential for fragmented or patchy forms of outcomes rather than a 'solid body' of evidence.

Finally, community interventions are not costless. They normally require the direct investment of new resources but may also involve redirecting existing resources away from other uses. It is thus important that evaluation not only shows what works, but at what cost. Policy makers seek evidence of an intervention's cost, as well as its effectiveness: is it an efficient use of scarce resources? How cost-effective is it compared with alternative ways of pursuing the same objectives? More generally, is it good value for money? In community interventions, such evidence is rarely provided. The discipline of economics defines resources as those things that contribute to the production of outputs – people, equipment, buildings and so on. Because resources are finite, there is a cost involved in committing them to one use in that benefits they could have achieved in another are sacrificed: the term 'opportunity cost' emphasises the concept of an opportunity foregone. It is clear that opportunity costs can be incurred even if no money is involved. Volunteers, for example, are not paid but the hours they devote to one project are not available for other voluntary tasks, hence their time is considered a cost of the project. Most interventions involve the use of dedicated resources that must be paid for: the Pembrokeshire SHARP, for example, employed action researchers whose salaries, travel costs, and so on were paid from the project grant. At the same time, however, and as with most community interventions, SHARP also required inputs from individuals working for the local authority and other statutory agencies. Although their time wasn't paid for from the project grant, their involvement incurred opportunity costs since the hours they devoted to the intervention were not available for other duties.

Economics, however, is not just about costs – it is about the *relationship* between costs and effects. Since resource scarcity means that resource allocation choices are inescapable, economists argue that the criteria on which those choices are made should be made explicit. The main criterion used within economics is *efficiency*, which is concerned with ensuring that decisions are taken that maximise the benefit from available resources. On efficiency grounds, therefore, one intervention cannot be preferred to another solely because it is less costly or solely because it is more effective – the decision must involve both (Drummond et al, 2005).

Clearly, different approaches to research on impact, effectiveness and cost are required if the evaluation of community-based approaches to health development is to avoid being seen as 'mission impossible'.

Evidence: what do we know and how do we know it?

Evidence is a notoriously ambiguous term. At its simplest, evidence provides grounds for a belief or theory, or information helping to establish the probability or likelihood of a proposition (Upshur, 2001). Yet many researchers freely acknowledge that what constitutes evidence is determined in large part by the knowledge community to which one belongs, and by what counts as acceptable knowledge within that community (Nutbeam, 1999; Lincoln, 2002). The basis for knowledge generation in participatory forms of evaluation, for example (which often uses an action research approach), contrasts sharply with that of the more traditional 'scientific' quantitative evaluation. The latter aims for the direct application of findings derived from research designed to produce statistically significant results across multiple sites. The former allows for abstraction of learning, to inform policy and practice elsewhere, through the development and refinement of theory, that is, beliefs about what works and why.

The favoured form of evidence is important because commissioners of services, if they apply evidence at all in their purchasing, will utilise research that fits with their preconception of what is acceptable and may neglect other types of evidence seen as less credible or rigorous. SHARP's commissioners in the Welsh Assembly Government were unusual in their openness to alternative forms of evidence. The problem with paying exclusive attention to 'rigorous' and 'robust' approaches in judging what counts as evidence is that it risks obscuring the theories, ideologies, values and principles that underpin any form of health intervention, although these strongly influence what gets accepted as valid evidence (Raphael, 2000). Lay forms of knowledge and expertise – the 'indigenous proficiencies' of community partners (Ansari et al, 2002) – tend to be invisible within the evidence-based movement and make scant contribution to what is seen to count as evidence.

The movement for evidence-based policy and practice in health*care* has utilised a hierarchical model of evidence, quantitative in approach and favouring experimental designs; randomised controlled trials (RCTs) and syntheses of their findings are placed at the top of the hierarchy. In this framework, qualitative and/or participatory methods tend to be understood as an early-phase aid to developing understanding of an intervention and its possible effects. This is difficult to reconcile with those who argue that a trials-based approach has limited usefulness in evaluating health *promotion* or other complex community-based initiatives. The World Health Organization, for example, has suggested that

> the use of randomised controlled trials to evaluate health promotion initiatives is, in most cases, inappropriate, misleading and unnecessarily expensive. (WHO, 2003, p 2)

Participation, the use of multiple methods, the goal of capacity building and appropriateness of method have all been suggested as principles that should underpin the evaluation of community health promotion initiatives, in order to accommodate their complex nature and potential long-term impact (WHO, 2003). It has been suggested that this shift in evaluation framework reflects

> the growing disillusionment, at a number of levels, with approaches to evaluation derived from methodologies that originated in the natural sciences. (WHO, 2003, p 263)

Participatory forms of research, on the other hand, argue both for the recapture of knowledge that has been excluded from conventional forms of inquiry, and for the redundancy of the conventional power structure between researcher and researched. Rather than treating research participants as mere repositories of data from which the researcher can extract relevant pieces of information, participatory research views the relationship between inquiry and participant as democratic, mutual and reciprocal.

Because it is difficult to specify a 'right' way of implementing or evaluating community health initiatives, it becomes problematic to specify an absolute form of evidence. However, despite the failure of traditional methods to supply evidence concerning effectiveness in the area of community-based health promotion initiatives, many still argue against more pluralistic, participatory approaches on the grounds of scientific rigour, generalisability, validity of results and replicability (Susman and Evered, 1978). For example, although a review of action research concluded that this approach should be considered as complementary to other research approaches in healthcare, concerns were raised over the quality of some research carried out within this paradigm, and over the lack of an agreed framework for evaluating its quality (Waterman et al, 2001).

Overall, while reviews of studies of effectiveness highlight the difficulties of evaluating complex community-based health promotion interventions, they generally come to similar conclusions: that there is a need for more rigorous methods for evaluation; that methods need to be appropriate to their setting; and that quantitative, trial-based, outcome-focused methods are seldom likely to be appropriate or provide the understanding necessary for generalising findings without including measures of process and qualitative data concerning meaning and the views of stakeholders.

Pluralistic approaches to evaluation (using multiple methods) hold promise as this involves using different forms of evidence from a variety of sources in order to evaluate an initiative. Beattie (1995) describes this as compiling a 'portfolio of evidence' detailing the processes and events that take place during and as a consequence of the community project. Qualitative information derived from interviews and observations can be combined with statistical data and documentary evidence in describing the change process. Although it may remain difficult to specify cause-and-effect relationships within the intervention, the emphasis on process and on community members and participants' perceptions and interpretations makes their detection more likely (Speller et al, 1997).

This is one reason why the search for evidence may need to focus on what types of change community health interventions are trying to achieve, which may include influencing services or changing social conditions. Action research not only attempts to counter the powerful currency of academic research by valuing the contribution that local people can make to the shared development of knowledge, but also develops that knowledge to inform action and construct evidence.

Evaluating SHARP: knowledge and learning as evidence

Evaluation is an important aspect of the SHARP initiative, built in at various levels within and across projects. The SHARP commissioners required each project to conduct an overall evaluation of their work, in addition to the reflective component of the action research cycle. The commissioners expected internal evaluation to provide examples of effective (and ineffective) practice in addressing health determinants so as to inform future policy development and practice, and evidence of enhanced potential for the further development of the participating communities or groups. Two years into the programme, an overarching evaluation was commissioned, to assess the overall effectiveness of the initiative against its main aims. Driven by different purposes, the internal and overarching levels of evaluation have taken different approaches.

The seven SHARP projects used different approaches to evaluation. The Barefoot, Holway, Right 2 Respect, BeWEHL (Bettws Women's Education, Health and Lifestyle) and Triangle projects all focused primarily on action – delivering a range of appropriate activities – with evaluation of these being a secondary objective. The HYPP (Health of Young People in Powys) project focused on evaluation (of various community development initiatives for young people), using action research, as its primary purpose. The Pembrokeshire SHARP project had also planned to use action research as an evaluation tool. Faced with challenging circumstances and comparatively slender resources, this project experienced tensions between developing action, conducting research and evaluating both.

Evaluation 'from within': the Pembrokeshire experience

The internal evaluation of the Pembrokeshire SHARP project tested the feasibility of developing a 'healthy living approach' in communities – without substantial external financial resources – and, by doing so, tested the feasibility of some important contemporary policy assumptions about what community health development and partnership work can deliver. The Pembrokeshire SHARP worked with community forums in three marginal communities: two acknowledged as relatively deprived, and one isolated by its rurality.

The participatory evaluation of the project's community health development approach and the action research process included a mix of quantitative and qualitative methods. In line with the 'portfolio of evidence' approach (Beattie, 1995), data were gathered from existing documents (including policy documents and minutes of meetings), diaries and reflective accounts, one-to-one and group interviews, postal questionnaires, and costing proformas. Evaluation questions focused on perceived outcomes (from the perspectives of community members, forum members and partners from statutory organisations); the process of implementation; and costs involved. This approach aimed to identify some key features – positive and negative – of using action research in a community initiative.

The evaluation found that many forum members and statutory service representatives expressed **faith in the process**: "Robust representations of issues in the communities because of the action research methods" (statutory sector representative on steering group).

However, the engagement of community members in research was hampered by **scepticism** about/fatigue with research, and by the language of 'professional' partners: "I could not see what benefits to the community at large it was going to have ... a lot of money was being spent on paying researchers instead of action in the community" (community forum member).

There were some **difficulties of matching expectations about project progress** across funders, academic partners, statutory sector partners and community representatives, as progress appeared slow, to some. Nevertheless, the Pembrokeshire evaluation suggested that, because of its underlying principle of participation, the action research approach allowed the views and priorities of a wide range of participants to be included: "I went to one meeting and there were 50 people there and people actually active in that meeting" (community forum member).

Yet doubts were still raised concerning the attribution of change to the project: "I want to believe that it will make a difference in some way, but I'm not actually sure how, and that's a very hard thing to say" (statutory sector representative).

Capacity building was perceived to be a key feature of the action research approach. Many positive comments were made by local participants: "I've learnt things but then I've had to do things that I wouldn't normally have done" (community researcher and forum member).

Moreover, benefits to local residents through their involvement with the project were also felt to have **enhanced engagement with the wider community**: "We've become a community and we've had community events, you know, which have brought people together and, in a sense, a lot of the problems that people had were tied in with loneliness and stress and.... I think those sort of things have been met in a different way, by just meeting together and having events" (community forum member).

Some concern was raised, however, about limitations in the skills acquired, leading to an impact on the quality of data gathered. Doubts notwithstanding, the community-based action research process enabled the **communication of local priorities, in an 'acceptable' language and format**, leading to more credibility with those in a position to influence service delivery and planning. It appeared that senior managers involved were actually more comfortable with the presentation of findings through reports or other formal media than the more usual means of community consultation, which sometimes involved heated and emotional public encounters.

The internal evaluation of the Pembrokeshire SHARP project suggests that a multi-strand approach to evaluation can produce useful evidence both on the process and perceived outcomes of the project. The risk of bias attached to gathering 'insider' views (as opposed to 'independent' or 'objective' views) is reduced by bringing in multiple viewpoints of all stakeholders. This in turn allows for a comparison to be made between the sometimes contradictory viewpoints of the different partners.

A comparative approach to evaluating SHARP

Recognising the difficulty of assessing the effectiveness of a programme delivered across seven diverse projects, programme funders commissioned an overarching evaluation of SHARP. The aim of this work, conducted by a separate evaluation team, was to assess SHARP's success in delivering key aims and objectives in the short and medium (and potentially long) term. The overarching evaluation was expected to contribute to evidence of the effectiveness of an action research approach from a comparative rather than a single-project perspective. The evaluation team saw its main aim as understanding how and why SHARP projects introduced particular forms of health action, the effects achieved within the communities involved, and the processes by which those outcomes were realised.

One of the main criticisms of conventional evaluation methods, when applied to community-level interventions, is the tendency to overlook or ignore the theoretical basis of the intervention. The assumptions that underpin every programme, whether articulated or not, may be viewed as a 'black box', leading to a focus on rigorous evaluation design, input and results, rather than on the processes that develop within the intervention and that may challenge the original thinking (Riley et al, 2005). In developing a comparative approach to evaluating SHARP, the evaluation team drew on the ideas of recent, theory-based approaches to evaluation (Weiss, 1995; Pawson and Tilley, 1997). These take for granted that all health and/or social programmes are based on explicit or implicit 'theories' about what is believed will work in producing hoped-for outcomes. Theories used in this sense are not remote abstractions but common-sense, practical ideas and beliefs.

Theory-based evaluation stresses that theories underpinning any initiative should be spelt out with the evaluators during the earliest stages, so participants understand their overall goals and can specify how to achieve these. Project theories become the 'test' by which projects are evaluated. However, when the evaluators began work some projects were already engaged in revising their original thinking, on the basis of their experience. In other cases, those who had written project proposals were no longer involved, or the circumstances in which projects were working had changed. This meant that individuals recruited to develop and implement the proposals could find themselves with unworkable or inappropriate models for community-level research or action or both. In such uncertain conditions it was difficult for project participants to specify their theories about what would work and why.

These conditions of uncertainty (arguably an inherent feature of community-level action research) led the team to take responsibility for articulating project theories, partly on the basis of project documentation and partly on the basis of knowledge generated through prolonged and extensive contact with the projects. They used a number of evaluation research methods, combining participant observation, semi-structured interviews and ad hoc conversations with analyses of project documentation, reports and so on. In all, they conducted over 60 visits to the projects over three years, spending time with project managers, partner organisations, action researchers and community participants, and observing their activities, in order to learn about the approaches taken locally, and how these worked in practice. This enabled them to track progress, observe and document the processes involved and, in many cases, to act as independent witness to support (or moderate) claims made by participants.

Using a combination of fieldwork and projects' own documentation, analyses and assessments of projects' progress and achievements were 'tested' through the construction of descriptive case studies, submitted to each project for scrutiny and discussion. In the case studies, the evaluation team sought to articulate the principles, values and beliefs that appeared to have shaped particular choices made by SHARP participants, to explain how participants had engaged with and actively interpreted the programme, and to generate a shared understanding of what counted as success at local level.

Although the 'ideal' models of theory-based evaluation tend to focus on prospective theorising with programme participants, the evaluation team found that the development of a theory-focused approach to evaluating community-based action research required the combination of prospective, contemporaneous and retrospective theorising. The overarching evaluation depended on working closely *with* the projects, acting as 'critical friends' on a joint evaluation journey focused on learning what works and for whom. The framework below was developed as a means of illustrating the ways in which 'theories' operated across the diversity of SHARP projects, that is, how participants made sense of and responded to the programme's ambitious aims. The framework illustrates how projects' 'theories' span different stages and operate at different levels of intervention, from planning, through implementation, to assessment of how and why the chosen approach worked, or not. Such theories are important forms of learning about what works, or not, and why – key questions for any evaluation, particularly one with a strong focus on learning, such as SHARP.

- The main reasonings, assumptions, values and beliefs underpinning each project were encapsulated in funding bids describing their action research plans and outcomes. Because of the short timescale for bid development and submission, those involved tended to be professional practitioners from a range of disciplines and organisations. These initial assumptions, which drew on participants' existing knowledge of the world, are described as projects' **underpinning theories**.

- **Working theories** developed through the processes of implementing action research and developing partnerships with a community or group. Because they reflect participants' developing but uncertain knowledge, working theories can feel tentative, particularly if they seem at odds with key assumptions contained in original proposals.

- **Emergent theories** appear at advanced stages of action research. They show how projects have made sense of the tensions (and potential dissonance) between planning, process and practice. Emergent theories thus reflect confidence in learning about what works (or not) in a particular context. This level of theory is based on the combined research and practitioner knowledge that informed original proposals; the practical experience gained through turning those ideas and concepts into a workable project at community level; the processes of reflecting on and evaluating the work; and the evidence generated. Through their emergent theories, project participants articulate what the longer-term legacy of their work is most likely to be. Emergent theories can then become the underpinning theories for a new cycle of developing, implementing and evaluating initiatives to further inform practice and policy.

An illustration of project theory in the Right 2 Respect (R2R) project, based in Wrexham youth service, is given in the box below. The key point here is that 'theory' is not a remote abstraction but is closely grounded in, and helps to explain, a project's chosen forms of practice in its own context.

Right 2 Respect: project theories

One of the **underpinning theories** found in the R2R project's proposal was that young women would be willing to take part in activities with an explicit focus on health (and an implicit focus on sexual health). A second theory reasoned that successful gender-specific work would require a commitment to acting on young women's priorities. These two theories are not necessarily commensurable, though they shared an assumption that a young women's project should reduce the chances of poor health/social exclusion. A third theory was that an action research approach would, if successful in improving the development and delivery of services, be assimilated by youth workers outside the project.

The tension between the first two theories has been resolved through the development of an important **working theory**, which suggests that the second of the above assumptions has greater validity. During implementation, the core team delivering the project found that, in order to engage young women in action research, their priorities had to come first and the focus on health had to be moderated. Because grounded in experience, this assessment is both more holistic and more personalised than original assumptions about what would work, and how. It is important to note, however, that the first theory has not been invalidated but rather successfully adapted to context.

The third underpinning theory outlined above proved less well founded. While R2R's action research work with young women has been successful, other youth workers viewed the team as a valuable external resource, rather than a source of learning on which to draw in developing good practice.

One of the project's **emergent theories** is that work on developing young women's skills and confidence is limited when conducted in a social vacuum: young men remain an important influence on young women's lives. As young men may benefit from the gender-specific approach, it needs to be extended to them. This, together with the observation that youth workers required more training and support before an action research approach could be widely adopted, led to the development of a gender-specific training programme in youth work. Thus, the gradual accumulation of learning and the development of new forms of practice enabled project leaders to reflect on and modify some key original assumptions, and influence mainstream service provision in ways likely to sustain longer-term change.

Similar examples of action research learning can be found across other SHARP projects. Although the reflexive, iterative and uncertain character of participatory community-based action research can make it difficult for participants to specify outcomes from the work at early stages, the action research approach encouraged constant reflection on how initiatives were progressing, whether they were working, and what might need to change. The theory-focused approach to evaluation, using the framework described earlier, therefore proved appropriate to the diverse, dynamic and developmental nature of the community-level action research projects within SHARP, where simple cross-project comparisons could rarely be made. Our evaluation suggests that, as projects' *emergent* theories are based on practical experience and mutual learning between project teams and other participants, they may well provide a sounder basis for future policy and practice than the professionally informed theories outlined in original proposals.

Forms of evidence: knowledge and learning

Maintaining the distinction drawn above between data and evidence, we can describe the *data* gathered across SHARP as mainly 'hard' or 'soft', qualitative or quantitative in nature. *Evidence*, however – the accumulation, combination and packaging of different forms of learning and knowledge – can be described in a different way, according to whether it appears to be *tangible* (concrete, measurable in form), or *testamentary* (from the Latin *testari*, 'to bear witness'). Using this typology enables us to move beyond the notion of a hierarchy of evidence towards a grounded view of the multiple forms that evidence can take. The concepts of tangible and testamentary forms of evidence enable us to distinguish between different, but equally important types of learning across SHARP that result from the construction and integration of different types of knowledge at local level. Both tangible and testamentary forms of evidence are important because they are related to different types of learning not adequately conveyed by the conventional distinction between quantitative and qualitative data.

Tangible forms of evidence

Tangible forms of evidence are positive in that they tell us what has been achieved in a visible or observable form: they exist as concrete phenomena. They include key outputs, in the form of action research products such as the published findings from local health needs surveys, dedicated toolkits developed for particular groups or populations, or training programmes and accredited qualifications developed during the life of projects. They also include tangible outcomes, such as new local initiatives or activities, impacts and effects on existing services, and broader community environmental improvements. Figure 7.1 gives some examples from SHARP.

Evidence from community-based action research evidence is often *embodied* rather than *abstract* in form: in themselves, participants can be living and breathing arguments for what projects have achieved. There are numerous examples across SHARP. In the Holway House project, for example, a local resident who developed diabetes was motivated to attend a smoking cessation course at the house, seek advice on healthy eating to lose weight, and train to become a lead walker in the Walk Your Way to Health initiative, now running weekly walks

Figure 7.1: Tangible forms of evidence in SHARP

Observable outcomes		Measurable outcomes	
New activities/ interventions: healthy eating and exercise projects, activities aimed at young people, women etc (Barefoot, Triangle, Holway)	Impact on services: development/ changes in service delivery, eg young people's influence on youth services (HYPP, R2R)	Community information: surveys, needs analysis, formal reports, action plans etc (Pembrokeshire)	Formal qualifications (BeWEHL); training courses/programmes, eg Open College Network in community research (Pembrokeshire), Higher National Certificate in gender-based youth work (R2R), participatory research/evaluation courses (Triangle)

Environmental improvements, eg CCTV and fewer void houses (Holway); skateboard park in Llanwrtyd Wells (HYPP)

Action guides: HYPPs OASIS Toolkit, Pembrokeshire's Community Researcher Handbook

from the estate. Similarly, a volunteer youth worker has been able to undertake a professional qualification and is now employed by youth services. A young mother who completed a computer course at the house and attended mum and toddler sessions is now employed by Sure Start to run the sessions and has begun training as a nursery nurse. Several residents have learned to drive, receiving free driving lessons in exchange for weekly voluntary work. Although such achievements are visible and measurable, the real health outcomes from this type of work tend to be 'soft': in the project worker's words, "all have gained independence and self-confidence and learned the value of commitment". Soft outcomes do not have to be invisible, however: Holway participants' increased self-confidence has been observed on multiple occasions. Some have, for example, spoken at a number of dissemination events over five years and, on one occasion, confidently and publicly defended their project from would-be detractors.

Testamentary forms of evidence

Testamentary forms of evidence, on the other hand, can be categorised as 'witness statements': they can either tell us directly about what action research means, to participants and observers, or enable us to reasonably infer such meaning, and suggest avenues for further research exploration. Although qualitative in form, they work to provide *insight* rather than necessarily being capable of standing up to the form of intense analytic scrutiny to which conventional types of qualitative data are routinely subjected. Figure 7.2 illustrates how testamentary forms of evidence may draw on a wide range of information, including participants' and stakeholders' direct experiences of participatory processes, their views and opinions, and can include anecdotes and stories. This kind of evidence may contain process information, revealing positives *and* negatives about what has been learned and achieved, and how. It is capable of indicating immediate effects on participants and short- to mid-term impacts, potentially enables us to infer longer-term outcomes, and indicates where to look for further substantiating evidence. The 'personal testaments' of community participants can be particularly powerful statements of effect.

Testamentary forms of evidence bear witness to indicators of change at the community or individual level. For example, many of the short

Figure 7.2: Testamentary forms of evidence in SHARP

Outcome information: statements about what has changed/been achieved. What this means for participants and, potentially, others in terms of policy and practice, eg the need to view 'health' as 'wellbeing' in order to act on local priorities, and the need to build capacity at agency, as well as community, level.

Anecdotes/stories: used in pointed ways to illustrate evidence of change, suggest meaning/import, and infer future potential. Indicators of where to look for further evidence.

Process information: perceptions of participation, partnership and action research, based on direct personal experience or informed observation, eg difficulties of partnership work, time taken to engage any type of community; improved sense of control, skills, confidence within local people; building forms of social capital.

statements from Holway residents to the action researcher about how their estate had improved as a result of SHARP funding Holway House referred to the benefits for the whole community – more opportunities for people to get together, more things for people (especially young people) to do. Others, however, suggest an intensity of impact at the individual level. One community respondent, for example, claimed that "the house is our life. We had no life before the house". Anecdotes can similarly act as micro-forms of evidence, vehicles for conveying powerful instances of learning and experience. For example, during the external evaluators' survey of stakeholders, a respondent speaking about the Triangle project recounted a brief story of change. She recalled that a woman from one of the disadvantaged communities, who had never cooked a meal for her family because she lacked both knowledge and confidence, was able to cook a Christmas dinner for her extended family after taking part in the project's healthy eating/cooking initiative.

The first point to make is that we need to understand the power of anecdotes to those who recount them: they are told specifically because they reveal something on which the teller has reflected and come to view as important, and others are expected to understand that importance. Second, in only a few words they may reveal a great deal about the depth of disadvantage and need being addressed in some communities. Third, they can indicate what should be taken as success, in the local context. 'Anecdotes' can encapsulate learning and thus deserve greater recognition rather than being routinely dismissed as unacceptable (because non-generalisable) forms of evidence. They are instances of the specific, the particular and possibly the unique, but they are also good indicators of areas that deserve further research exploration. For example, the manager of the 'Barefoot' Health Workers project, speaking to the external evaluators, reported that:

> "There is an elusiveness and slipperiness to the 'facts' collected from the three [BME] communities. The *evidence* (especially the anecdotal/in passing/reflective) is an attempt to understand aspects of the communities – their perceptions/concerns – and to help to see if these really are closely matched to the centrally determined health promotion agenda, or whether we are simply running two worlds in parallel which just happen to sit comfortably around a common initiative. Getting a handle on this is important if the project and other public health initiatives are going to succeed in the long run."

This also raises the broader question of who decides what the evidence means in any particular context. Project leaders and project workers may, for example, place quite different interpretations on the same piece of evidence – 'two worlds running in parallel'. This is an issue of power that relates, in part, to who *speaks for* a project, whose voice renders the account. Where multiple voices tell a similar story about a project, we may, for example, feel greater certainty about the validity of that story than when we hear different, competing versions. This returns us to the point made above – that participatory approaches to research value the knowledge of local people (and practitioners). Yet we also need to understand that many community participants may have little interest in the formal, written presentation of evidence, viewing this as an arcane (and probably dull) activity best left to 'experts'. In the Pembrokeshire SHARP, for example, despite sterling efforts from the action researchers to engage community representatives in writing reports on the work, local people remained adamant that this was not their role.

In the Holway project, the lead researcher suggested that:

> If residents are to be effective in partnership with the county council and other agencies, they will need to be well-informed about policy, and able to write documents supported with evidence. This requires skills that are not general in the population and it is the ability of what Holway people see as 'the men in suits' to write such documents that keeps the ordinary citizen at a disadvantage. (Moore, 2005, p 34)

We now turn from considering the types of learning, knowledge and evidence that derived from the community-based action research approach across SHARP, and some of the challenges in providing such evidence, to the more difficult 'so what?' question. SHARP was designed, from inception, to influence national and local policy and practice. What is the potential for evidence from comparatively small-scale but successful community-based action research programmes to exert such influence?

From evidence to influence

SHARP projects have amassed knowledge about different forms of practice that may well be transferable to other contexts. There is ample evidence of learning across projects, packaged as evidence through formal reports and other means of dissemination, in order to convince and influence others. Much of the evidence from SHARP provides a window on to the wider determinants of health and wellbeing. Projects have worked to translate a policy focus on 'health inequalities' into a set of practical commitments to articulating and acting on local priorities. Action research rejects the traditional research view of non-academic participants as repositories from which data can be extracted and so the evidence generated is firmly grounded in local understandings and practices. This method of inquiry has proven to be challenging, in part because the understandings of 'health' found in SHARP are broad, but also because projects' work has implications for policy makers, practitioners from a wide range of disciplines, and service-providing organisations, at local and national level.

What constitutes evidence is governed not only by the rigour and appropriateness of methods and reporting or the persuasive power of participants' testaments, but also by the political and 'favoured knowledge' environment of policy makers and service commissioners and by the specific policy hooks on to which evidence can be attached. Although we now work in a political climate where the problem of social inequalities in health is not only openly acknowledged but has received much policy attention, barriers still remain. As SHARP projects sought to explain what they had achieved and what they had learned to policy makers, it became clear that evidence from community-based action research projects can be rubbished and rejected, or just ignored, on 'scientific' grounds as an insufficiently rigorous method. This is because such accounts may be seen as subjective, presented by individuals as explanations of how the project has started to change their lives rather than as a set of statistics. They may also be rejected on the grounds that numbers of participants or outcomes are too small to permit statistical tests of reliability. Conversely, there was evidence of acceptance of data from the projects that did have the right sort of stamp or pedigree – survey results, for example.

However, as Weiss (2001) reminds us, evidence is not the only contender for influence. Despite widespread calls for 'evidence-based' policy and practice, other forms of knowledge, including personal experience and political considerations, guide public health and social policy decisions. The influence of research on policy and practice is also likely to be tempered by factors such as financial constraints and shifting timescales (Elliott and Popay, 2000); indeed, these influences were observed and experienced as community needs assessments and housing surveys were reported in the SHARP projects. Moreover, different kinds of evidence are not always commensurable; practical judgement is needed if they are to be used effectively and widely.

Health promotion practitioners sometimes argue that a wholesale shift in favour of the acceptability of evidence derived from participatory, community-based research knowledge may be all that is needed to develop improved services and more informed policies (Hills and Mullett, 2000; Raphael, 2000; Tones, 2002). Evaluators, however, point to a more complex reality, where 'evidence' performs multiple functions for policy makers, providing them with data, ideas and arguments on which they draw, selectively, according to their own political and ideological preferences (Weiss, 1991). Evidence can also be used as political ammunition, or to lace policy making with the appearance of rationality (Booth, 1988). The ways that policies are developed, implemented, monitored and revised are always shaped by the wider social and political context (Shaxson, 2005) and the significance of the social and political context in which knowledge is produced and evidence deployed remains under-appreciated (Stone et al, 2001).

Those potentially on the receiving end of the evidence (and thus the target for particular arguments, ideas, recommendations and so on) cannot be viewed as empty vessels waiting to be filled with information before taking policy and/or practice decisions. This is where different forms of expertise and evidence are likely to find common ground or, potentially, hostile territory. The usefulness of evidence generated through the various forms of knowledge produced through action research remains contingent on key public sector agencies' and policy makers' capacity and willingness to learn from, and be convinced by, the product. Ideas, tested and shown to be feasible, can suddenly become 'best practice' where an initiative needs models that 'fit' to display. Women-only swimming classes fitted well with a policy commitment to free access to community swimming pools and with broader social inclusion measures under a banner of social justice. Although the spread of particular initiatives may be helped by recognition as a 'best practice', the process of working the initiative through and building it as a partnership can easily become lost in translation. The wider test of a responsive, inclusive process of service development – the local version of action research – is perhaps not sufficiently tangible or graspable.

According to the preferences, perceptions and values of recipients, the status of evidence may shift between recognition, acceptance and rejection. For example, in a telephone survey of stakeholders across SHARP conducted by the overarching evaluation team, the question of whether their local project was 'value for money' exercised a number of respondents. For some, projects were resource-intensive and expensive ways of working with communities and groups, because of the small numbers of beneficiaries. For others, however, the depth of need addressed and the positive outcomes for participants and agencies represented a sound return on investment. These different views are unlikely to be solved by appeals solely to 'evidence', as they clearly involve value-based arguments and judgements. As O'Neill and Williams point out:

> As politics and policy become more concerned with 'evidence', the relationship between 'expert evidence' and political judgements and decisions becomes increasingly complicated. (O'Neill and Williams, 2004, p 38)

The usefulness and transferability of the evidence generated by the multiple participants in action research projects across SHARP may remain contingent on key public sector agencies' and policy makers' capacity to learn and their willingness to be persuaded by the arguments mounted. Some projects have had considerable success in influencing local agency policy and practice. In other projects, participants argue that their experience demonstrates that a long-term view is needed, where resources can be committed to disadvantaged communities without expecting early returns. Yet the contemporary context for most major service providers is one of instability, where organisational and policy change have become routine (while remaining stressful), and where resources for development work lie mainly within the (insecure) voluntary sector while short-term performance indicators (such as reducing NHS waiting lists) dominate statutory sector work. In this context, notions of 'evidence for change' may carry little weight unless such change is in line with core agency agendas.

Community participation and multisectoral partnership work are key mechanisms for change within a national policy framework of health improvement for the most disadvantaged communities, but policy makers and service providers at local level may still find these unfamiliar and uncomfortable concepts. Getting partnership and participation into practice requires a synthesis of radically different cultures and philosophies about how people and organisations learn and change. Ironically, willingness to learn from evidence provided by initiatives like SHARP could benefit professional practitioners charged with responsibility for improving health and other services aimed at the community, because of their insight into community priorities and their examples of effective practice in community engagement in work on the broader determinants of health and wellbeing.

Yet it seems likely that community-based health programmes based on genuine consultation and participation will remain difficult to place among the core demands of major agencies' work. Not surprisingly, perhaps, there still seems to be both a lack of understanding, among statutory agencies, of the links between community-based activities to promote wellbeing and broader outcomes/longer-term impacts on health, and a reluctance to invest in such programmes until the evidence base is perceived as 'stronger' (that is, more quantitative). Building capacity *within agencies* to work more effectively with communities remains a problem that cannot simply be resolved by calls for 'better' evidence.

References

Beattie, A. (1995) 'Evaluation in community development for health: an opportunity for dialogue', *Health Education Journal*, vol 54, no 4, pp 465-72.

Booth, T. (1988) *Developing Policy Research*, Aldershot: Gower.

Chelimsky, E. (1997) 'Thoughts for a new evaluation society', Evaluation, vol 3, no 1, pp 97-118.

Cohen, A.P. (1985) *The Symbolic Construction of Community*, London: Routledge & Kegan Paul.

Coote, A., Allen, J. and Woodhead, D. (2004) *Finding out What Works: Building Knowledge about Complex, Community-based Initiatives*, Policy Paper, London: King's Fund.

Drummond, M.F., Sculpher, M.J., Torrance, G.W., O'Brien, B.J. and Stoddardt, G.L. (2005) *Methods for the Economic Evaluation of Health Care Programmes* (3rd edn), Oxford: Oxford University Press.

El Ansari, W., Phillips, C.J. and Zwi, A.B. (2002) 'Narrowing the gap between academic professional wisdom and community lay knowledge: perceptions from partnerships', *Public Health*, vol 116, no 3, pp 151-9.

Elliot, H. and Popay, J. (2000) 'How are policy makers using evidence? Models of research utilisation and local NHS policy making', *Journal of Epidemiology and Community Health*, vol 54, no 6, pp 461-8.

Hepworth, J. (1997) 'Evaluation in health outcomes research: linking theories, methodologies and practice in health promotion', *Health Promotion International*, vol 12, no 3, pp 233-8.

Hills, D. (2004) *Evaluation of Community-level Interventions for Health Improvement: A Review of Experience in the UK*, London: Health Development Agency (www.hda.nhs.uk).

Hills, M. and Mullett, J. (2000) 'Community-based research: creating evidence-based practice for health and social change', Paper presented at the Qualitative Evidence-based Practice Conference, Coventry University, 15-17 May.

Jewkes, R. and Murcott, A. (1998) 'Community representatives: representing the "community"?', *Social Science & Medicine*, vol 46, no 6, pp 843-58.

Labonte, R. (2001) 'Advocacy: from setting the agenda to enabling the actors', *Promotion & Education*, vol 2, pp 35-6 (Special Edition of the *International Journal of Health Promotion and Education*).

Lincoln, Y. (2002) 'On the nature of qualitative evidence', Paper presented at the Annual Meeting of the Association for the Study of Higher Education, Sacramento, CA, 21-24 November.

Moore, R. (2005) *Final Report of the Holway Project*, Liverpool: University of Liverpool.

Morgan, L.N. (2001) 'Community participation in health: perpetual allure, persistent challenge', *Health Policy and Planning*, vol 16, no 3, pp 221-30.

Nutbeam, D. (1999) 'The challenge to provide evidence in health promotion', *Health Promotion International*, vol 14, no 2, pp 99-101.

O'Neill, M. and Williams, G. (2004) 'Community and agency engagement in an action research study in South Wales', *Critical Public Health*, vol 14, no 1, pp 37-47.

Pawson, R. and Tilley, N. (1997) *Realistic Evaluation*, London: Sage Publications.

Raphael, D. (2000) 'The question of evidence in health promotion', *Health Promotion International*, vol 15, no 4, pp 355-67.

Rifkin, S. (1996) 'Paradigms lost: toward a new understanding of community participation in health programmes', *Acta Tropica*, vol 61, no 2, pp 79-92.

Riley, T., Hawe, P. and Shiell, A. (2005) 'Contested ground: how should qualitative evidence inform the conduct of a community intervention trial?', *Journal of Health Services Research & Policy*, vol 10, no 2, pp 103-10.

Robinson, G.H. and Hill, J. (1995) 'Problems in the evaluation of community-wide initiatives' in J.P. Connell, A.C. Kubish, L.B. Schorr and C.H. Weiss (eds) *New Approaches to Evaluating Community Initiatives. Volume 1: Concepts, Methods and Contexts*, Washington, DC: Aspen Institute.

Shaxson, L. (2005) 'Is your evidence robust enough? Questions for policy makers and practitioners', *Evidence & Policy*, vol 1, no 1, pp 101-11.

Shediac-Rizkallah, M.C. and Bone, L.R. (1998) 'Planning for the sustainability of community-based health programs: conceptual frameworks and future directions for research, practice and policy', *Health Education Research: Theory and Practice*, vol 13, no 1, pp 87-108.

Speller, V., Learmonth, A., and Harrison, D. (1997) 'The search for evidence of effective health promotion', *British Medical Journal*, vol 315, pp 361-3.

Stone, D., Maxwell, S. and Keating, M. (2001) 'Bridging research and policy', Paper presented at an international workshop funded by the UK Department for International Development, Radcliffe House, Warwick University, 16-17 July.

Susman, G.I. and Evered, R.D. (1978) 'An assessment of the scientific merits of action research', *Administrative Science Quarterly*, vol 23, pp 582-602.

Tones, K. (2002) 'Evaluating health promotion: a tale of three errors', *Patient Education and Counselling*, vol 39, pp 227-36.

Upshur, R. (2001) 'The status of qualitative research as evidence', in J. Morse et al (eds) *The Nature of Qualitative Evidence*, London: Sage Publications.

Waterman, H., Tillen, D., Dickson, R. and de Konig, K. (2001) 'Action research: a systematic review and guidance for assessment', *Health Technology Assessment*, vol 5, no 23.

Weiss, C.H. (1991) 'Policy research: data, ideas, or arguments?', in P. Wagner, B. Wittrock and H. Wollmann (eds) *Social Sciences and Modern States: National Experiences and Theoretical Crossroads*, Cambridge: Cambridge University Press, pp 307-32.

Weiss, C.H. (1995) 'Nothing as practical as good theory: exploring theory-based evaluation for comprehensive community initiatives for children and families', in J.P. Connell, A.C. Kubish, L.B. Schorr and C.H. Weiss (eds) *New Approaches to Evaluating Community Initiatives. Volume 1: Concepts, Methods and Contexts*, Washington, DC: Aspen Institute.

Weiss, C.H. (2001) 'What kind of evidence in evidence-based policy?', Paper presented at the Third International, Inter-disciplinary Evidence-Based Policies and Indicator Systems Conference, Durham, 4-7 July (www.cemcentre.org/eg/2003/, accessed 11 July).

White, D.G. (2001) 'Evaluating evidence and making judgements of study quality: loss of evidence and risks to policy and practice decisions', *Critical Public Health*, vol 11, no 1, pp 3-17.

Wimbush, E. and Watson, J. (2000) 'An evaluation framework for health promotion: theory, quality and effectiveness', *Evaluation*, vol 6, no 3, pp 301-21.

WHO (World Health Organization) (2003) *Health Promotion Evaluation: Recommendations to Policy-makers. Report of the WHO European Working Group on Health Promotion*, Copenhagen: WHO.

Zakus, J.D. and Lysack, C.L. (1998) 'Revisiting community participation', *Health Policy and Planning*, vol 13, no 1, pp 1-12.

EIGHT

Social theory, social policy and sustainable communities

Robert Moore

Introduction: the 1998 White Paper

The 1998 White Paper *Better Health – Better Wales* (Welsh Office, 1998) addressed the issues that most directly affect the health of people in the Sustainable Health Action Research Programme (SHARP) areas. The White Paper recognised the social causes of ill health and also noted that while health in Wales was slowly improving from a low base, health inequalities persisted (§6.16). In proposing policies to address poor health in Wales, the White Paper specifically aimed to reduce health inequalities (§6.16, 7.10), although, as in England (Graham, 2004), resulting policy documents employed the term 'health inequalities' in a number of different ways.

The White Paper laid great stress on multidisciplinary collaborative and intersectoral approaches within the health services. It asserted that health services could not be engaged in health promotion by themselves and that social and physical environments also needed to be improved; that people need to feel safe from crime to be free from the anxieties that can undermine health and wellbeing (§3.11); and that good housing is essential for health (§5.3). Furthermore, people were more likely to be healthy in work that out of work (§3.5). Agencies working in the fields of health, education, criminal justice and the environment were not just to collaborate with one another, but were to form partnerships with local communities. Thus, the White Paper went beyond advocating an integrated health service: 'Long-term action is needed to tackle the root causes of health and economic inequality. This may mean a new approach to maintaining health and to using health and social care services as a community resource' (§3.4).

The idea of publicly provided services being a *resource* was innovative if not revolutionary. Since its inception, the NHS has been provider-led, but according to the White Paper, health authorities were to have 'duties of partnership' (§6.15) and health improvement programmes were to include locally determined priorities (§7.13), although *how* local is not stated. Chapter Six of the White Paper sets out a vision of partnership between a range of agencies and local communities, acting together to promote the health of the Welsh population. Forged in the euphoria of the founding of the Welsh Assembly and informed by the large body of research accumulated in medical studies and sociological research, the White Paper adopted a progressive approach to health and health service delivery. With the formation of the Welsh Assembly Government in 1998, the almost evangelical commitment to partnership and 'joined-up' policy making continued. The Assembly asserted in its 2001 paper *Improving Health in Wales* that health policy would encompass action to tackle the social causes of ill health and social action to sustain good health:

> The Assembly has developed – and is implementing – a number of strategies to counteract social exclusion and to create a *socially inclusive* Wales. It recognises the importance of building and supporting strong *communities* where the values of citizenship and collective action can grow. A new way of making and implementing policy has taken root and is being nurtured. Instead of the old practice of restricting the development of important policies to a relatively small group of experts in government, the new Wales is characterised by an *opening up* of the policy making process. This Plan builds on wide consultation over the elements that make it up and is part of the process of replacing elite policy making by *participative* policy development. Our policy here is to build on this commitment and to continue *to enhance the citizen's voice* at the heart of policy. (National Assembly for Wales, 2001a, p 5, emphasis in original)

In the same year, the Assembly announced its Communities First programme, which, while broader in its scope and geographical coverage, embodied similar ethics and politics to those found in the SHARP programme:

> The health promotion strategy's strong community focus means that it is coherent with the Assembly's approach to community strategies – working at the local authority level or wider – and *Communities First* working with smaller localities. Action will help to develop and expand the health improvement component of *Communities First* and community strategies. It will include the development of a

practical planning tool to help communities to benchmark their area against the core characteristics of a healthy community together with new guidance to help all parts of the NHS, but particularly Local Health Groups and primary care teams, to develop their work with communities. (National Assembly for Wales, 2001b, p 8)

A healthy population is also seen as necessary to a strong economy and the need to promote good health for economic reasons is stated most clearly in the November 2005 consultation document *Wales:A Vibrant Economy* (Welsh Assembly Government, 2005, p 7).

By 2006, much of the vision remained unrealised because from 1998 the issue of hospital waiting lists has overtaken all others in health policy. Wales in particular has a poor record on waiting lists. Constant press attention to the issue, with regular stories of individual suffering or family tragedies, countered with fresh government targets, diverted attention – and resources – from the goals of the White Paper. In meetings with SHARP participants, senior health officials stated their interest in the objectives of partnership and affirmed the value of locally defined priorities but expressed regret that their resources had to be devoted to reducing hospital waiting lists.

For social scientists, there are significant omissions from the White Paper. First, there was no direct reference to *inequality itself* as a cause of ill health as argued by Wilkinson (1996, 2005). The White Paper addresses inequality of income but almost exclusively as a correlate of ill health; poorer people are more likely to experience ill health and to die younger than average. This is conspicuously the case and the reasons are alluded to in the White Paper. But following Wilkinson, it must be said that social inequality increases ill health and early death for the whole Welsh population (but see Judge, 1995; Wilkinson, 1995; Gravelle, 1998). It is not the poor alone who suffer from the unequal distribution of income, wealth and material resources. We might expect therefore that reducing inequality should raise questions about the distribution of wealth and incomes and of redistribution, but these are on no political party's agenda. Since 'New' Labour came to power, there has nevertheless been some redistribution through the tax and benefits system that has removed 1.2 million children from poverty (Sutherland, 2000, p 16), but the effects of these policies may diminish over time (Brewer et al, 2006a, p 4) and the initial reforms also left one in five of the poorest children *worse* off (Sutherland and Piachaud, 2000, p 9). Poverty measured by household expenditure rather than income shows an increase in child poverty of nearly three per cent between 1996/97 and 2002/03 (Brewer et al, 2006b). The unwillingness of UK governments to confront questions of inequality and redistribution may be the reason why inequality as such is not addressed with any rigour in the White Paper, or in any other Welsh policy document. There is no action proposed 'to tackle the root causes of ... economic inequality' (§3.4). This omission continues in the Assembly's economic development consultation paper, which, while strong on *community* and *partnership* and hoping to address social exclusion, does not contain the words *inequality* or *redistribution* (Welsh Assembly Government, 2005).

The incoming New Labour administration in 1997 was not even prepared to consider redressing the upward redistribution from the poor to the rich through the tax and benefits systems that had been a feature of previous Conservative governments. For its part, the Welsh administration may share the commonly held World Bank belief that economic growth will not only benefit all, but also increase the share of national wealth enjoyed by the poorest. This would mean that if growth policies were pursued effectively, no action would be needed on equality. This belief is, regrettably perhaps, without foundation (Gordon, 2005).

The term *social exclusion* occurs only twice in the White Paper. In §3.20-3.22, it is used with reference to minority ethnic groups and rural populations. Social exclusion is also mentioned in the brief discussion of SHARP (§8.5). The Social Inclusion Unit is also referred to in stating the aim of breaking down barriers to collaboration at the heart of government in Wales. The omission is surprising, given the frequent references to social exclusion and inclusion in public debate and the fact that poor health is normally cited as one feature of social exclusion. People do not just happen to be in a state of exclusion, however; social exclusion is *a process* whereby certain social actors actively exclude others. This exclusion may be delivered in face-to-face relationships or it may be embodied in the routine operations of agencies ('institutionalised exclusion'). In the SHARP projects processes of social exclusion could be seen operating at very close quarters both in the encounters between local people and other actors and in the operation of the agencies and institutions in which these interpersonal relationships were embedded. The next section of this chapter will explore processes of social exclusion.

Social capital is not a concept that occurs specifically in the White Paper. This is a third surprising omission because it is an idea that has been the subject of an excellent review by the Social Exclusion Unit (SEU, 2001) and regularly features in social policy debates. Cabinet ministers in Westminster have discussed the promotion of social capital with prominent American social scientists and a social capital module is now included in the General Household Survey, so attempts are being made to measure it. Furthermore, questions on aspects of social capital have been included in the Health Education Monitoring Survey since 1998, a report by Boreham and colleagues (2000) in the *Health Survey for England 2000* and a report based on the British Household Panel Survey (Pevalin and Rose, 2003). The interest in social capital seems to lie mainly in governments' desire to find ways of shifting responsibilities for welfare and wellbeing from the state to the individual or the local community.

The White Paper only makes indirect reference to social capital in §3.14 by asserting that networks of families, friends and social institutions (for example, churches, clubs, sports facilities and voluntary organisations) can be important in developing self-esteem and confidence and in providing support. Interestingly, in discussing possible interventions in §3.17 it lists eight points directed to supporting or changing the behaviour of individuals and only two to building resources in the community; 'supporting youth and family groups at the community level' and 'encouraging community support networks'. We will explore the question of social capital below.

Social exclusion

Levitas (1996, 2000, 2006) asks whether social exclusion is a useful term. Is it simply a description of the consequences of, or even a euphemism for, poverty? The idea of exclusion was introduced by Peter Townsend in his 1979 description of poverty, whereby people 'are, in effect, excluded from ordinary living patterns, customs and activities' by poverty (1979, p 32). Poor people are thus 'shut out' from the mainstream; they cannot join in locally expected patterns of consumption, their children cannot go on school trips, they cannot afford visits to family and friends, or holidays. The idea highlights the non-material consequences of material deprivation. The Social Exclusion Unit defined social exclusion as 'a shorthand for what can happen when individuals or areas suffer from a combination of linked problems such as, unemployment, low skills, low incomes, poor housing, high crime environments, bad health and family breakdown' (SEU, 1997). This definition plainly underlies the problems that SHARP was meant to address. Restoring incomes, and overcoming poverty and ill health required a local approach to 'linked problems'. For many in the SHARP populations, economic recovery through employment would not be immediately possible because of low skill levels, poor health and, perhaps, a 'culture of poverty' in which adaptations to deprivation become maladaptive for rejoining the mainstream:

> The culture of poverty is both a reaction and an adaptation of the poor to their marginal position in a class stratified, highly individuated, capitalist society.... Once it comes into existence it tends to perpetuate itself from generation to generation because of its effects on the children. (Lewis, 1968, pp 5-6)

The problem of social exclusion creating the conditions for its own perpetuation was recognised in the Assembly's strategic framework for economic development (Welsh Assembly Government, 2005, p 73) but not elaborated on. The most recent and comprehensive study of social exclusion is the 2006 'millennium survey' *Poverty and Social Exclusion in Britain* (Pantazis et al, 2006). This study is based on interviews with individuals drawn from nearly 3,000 households. The data are therefore aggregate data that were analysed to provide an overview of poverty and exclusion in Britain. The SHARP projects were complementary to the more statistical analyses in providing the researchers with the opportunity to view people not through survey data but as real people living out their lives over a five-year period. While the academic researchers may not have seen their task in this way at the beginning of SHARP, it rapidly became clear that they were acquiring a detailed and privileged insight into social processes that had hitherto been largely (although not exclusively) studied through aggregate statistics. This was notably the case in those projects that were based on a 'community of location'.

Policy responses to exclusion may embody various 'discourses', of which Levitas explored three. The first is a redistributive discourse; 'the central problem is that the poor lack resources – not just money but also access to collectively provided services; poverty remains at the core' (Levitas, 2006, p 125). While government policies did not and do not countenance redistribution through progressive taxation, *Better Health – Better Wales* and the SHARP initiative embodied the need to achieve a degree of redistribution of publicly provided services towards the poorest. Levitas' second 'discourse', social exclusion as labour market exclusion, was an important element in all the SHARP projects and especially in locations where a substantial industrial base had collapsed. Industrial transformations were making old skills redundant and eliminating low-skilled jobs. Traditional men's occupations in the industrial sector were being replaced by service sector employment. In Flintshire – a 'booming' county – there was also a demand for skilled labour that could not be met locally. At the grass roots, labour market exclusion could not be overcome simply by advertising vacancies and providing training. The long-term impact of unemployment and more deeply rooted personal problems needed to be overcome; these include low levels of literacy, extremely low levels of self-confidence, low motivation and the impact of long-term labour market exclusion on domestic lives that become unsuited to the routines of a working life.

Getting people into training and employment is a central plank of government policy but it does not necessarily address the possibility of labour market inclusion exacerbating or creating health problems through highly subordinate and exploited roles that entail low pay, long hours and high levels of stress. Here, and especially in the case of minority ethnic groups, the form of social inclusion (or 'integration') may itself be the problem, although not one that would be recognised or accepted by government.

The 'moral underclass discourse' (Levitas' third) focuses on the moral deficiencies of the poor, their propensity to criminal and antisocial behaviour, and their lack of self-discipline and self-control represented by unmarried teenage mothers and absent teenage fathers. In Charles Murray's account of the underclass, they choose not to work (see Moore, 2001). The White Paper and SHARP did not adopt this approach to social exclusion but the existence of the discourse at the national level may have been deeply stigmatising for the populations included in SHARP. Furthermore, because the Holway and the Gurnos/Galon Uchaf estates in Merthyr Tydfil were seen as problem areas inhabited by problem people, local press reports focused on delinquency, crime and disorder in these areas. Longer established residents in Monkton in Pembrokeshire felt that the estate was becoming a ghetto where the council housed problem tenants. In the case of Gurnos/Galon Uchaf, its reputation is now enshrined in contemporary 'Welsh realist' fiction (Barry, 2002; Griffiths, 2001). Local residents and public officials frequently expressed views or displayed attitudes belonging to the 'moral underclass discourse' and the residents of these areas not only knew this to be the case, but also often experienced the attitudes in face-to-face encounters. Partnership was to become a means by which the local population was to collaborate with a range of agencies to reduce the crime and disorder that was blighting people's lives. Managing effective partnerships was one aspect of the development of social capital in the localities (see below) and another was the ability of residents to secure a more positive image of the estate in the local press.

Levitas was correct to ask whether social exclusion was a useful term. It is not useful when it is simply to avoid words like poverty and deprivation: '[Social exclusion] ... is a way of looking at the concept of poverty rather than an alternative to it' (Lister, 2004, p 74). The term is useful if it is not confused with poverty because it does describe an important dimension of poverty – namely, the extent to which poorer people are 'shut out' by their poverty. The term enables us to unpack the lived reality of poverty and to see multiple aspects of multiple deprivation. The idea of social exclusion also alerts us to agency in the creation of poverty and deprivation. People may be thought just to be poor, but if they are excluded someone has to be doing the exclusion. We might note in passing that some people choose to exclude themselves from 'the mainstream' – the super-rich on their country estates and the merely wealthy in their gated and guarded housing developments, for example – but there are no policies designed to reintegrate them and overcome their exclusion.

As Ruth Lister has noted, 'exclusion arises from the interplay of class, status and political power and serves the interests of the included' (Lister, 2004, p 77). So in the SHARP locations we must ask who is doing the excluding or how social exclusion is produced. At the institutional level, people are excluded by the operation of markets; they simply cannot afford certain consumer goods. The extent of their exclusion from consumption is reinforced by television advertising that constantly tells them that unaffordable goods and services are essential for a good life and perfect parenthood. Children are constantly urged to own or consume what other children are shown to have. This may further heighten family tensions and actually deepen poverty by encouraging parents to purchase clothing and other items for their children so that the latter will not be stigmatised and bullied by their peers. Market exclusion is also important for health. Few mothers can be unaware of what constitutes a healthy diet, but high-quality fresh fruit and vegetables (for example) may be inaccessible and unaffordable.

Residents may be excluded from accessing public services, not by poverty as such but by lack of public transport; for example, Holway residents could not attend evening courses at Deeside College. The Pembrokeshire SHARP locations also experienced communications problems. When the Department of Work and Pensions withdrew an outreach worker from the Holway project, the manager asserted that "if they want us, they know where we are", by which he meant that Holway residents could use public transport and take two buses each way on a round trip of 32 miles. Through SHARP, Holway residents gained the services of a dietician, who started a healthy eating session at the project house, but she was withdrawn as a result of a funding conflict between east and west Flintshire, a conflict internal to the health service to which Holway residents were not party. This, along with the closure of a breakfast club in a local secondary school through lack of funds, was an outcome quite contrary to the Assembly's stated intention of addressing the underlying causes of ill health in a joined-up way. A literacy course that was popular with young mothers could not be followed by the numeracy course they had requested because the funding regime set by central government did not allow the college to provide two consecutive courses in any one location. These were examples of public services not simply being inaccessible but *becoming* inaccessible (or less accessible) in the lifetime of the SHARP project – human beings with names and faces made decisions that excluded. Similar actors in central and local government are also to be found formulating policies that exclude, or, as in the case of the Child Support Agency, failing to implement policies. While it may be argued that the whole population of Wales lost out in changes or failures of service delivery – they were the 'collateral damage' of policy decisions – the fact remains that SHARP residents were in most need of these services.

In exploring social exclusion within small populations or communities, we should not lose sight of the overarching reality:

> To a substantial degree, what we now call social exclusion is the result of the failure of overstretched public services over the past two decades to maintain the vision of Beveridge and adapt it to a fast changing economy. Tight control of resources by the last government played a large part in denying effective services to poor areas. In many districts, services have been incrementally withdrawn from estates and poor neighbourhoods in order to achieve budget cuts. Even where services have been maintained, the increase in need consequent on growing joblessness and poverty has outstripped public services' capacity to provide. The outcome is that residents of poor areas have found it increasingly hard to access the public services they need; and very often the quality of those services is poor. (Page, 2000, p 102)

People also experience exclusion in face-to-face encounters. Many such examples were recounted by residents in the SHARP projects, most notably of dismissive and contemptuous attitudes on the part of counter staff in Flintshire council's housing department. One official discussing a deeply indebted Holway tenant threatened with eviction simply commented that the tenant 'should not have got into debt in the first place' without taking into consideration the effect of Working Families Tax Credit overpayments on the tenant's situation and the lack of advice services available to the tenant confronted with demands for repayment. Two local bank managers were approached by the Holway researchers to discuss Holway residents' problems in using local banking services – the problems were dismissed with comments such as, "There is no problem, this is the friendliest bank I have every worked in". Nevertheless, letters from the researchers asking to meet the bank managers to discuss these issues remained unanswered. A striking example of the way in which people can be drawn into adopting exclusionary attitudes even towards their peers was provided by a workman who, when asked whether there would be any local briefing about a CCTV system he was installing, replied: "All these people need to know is that they are being watched". Residents' sense of exclusion was at its deepest and most dispiriting in exchanges characterised by mutual incomprehension, when residents felt they were not being listened to. They were not themselves always very adept in presenting their own arguments and sometimes shouting at the 'suits' was their only strategy. At one meeting this gave rise to an incident where an official was heard to say to another, "Don't answer, they're not worth it", a comment that was long remembered in the Holway estate. Rejection and humiliation can be experienced within the health service itself; for example, residents reported that some GPs were quite transparent in their contempt for unemployed patients of working age. Whether the patients' perceptions were correct or not, the GPs were not considering how their demeanour might undermine the outcomes of their clinical activities.

The relative inability of people to overcome social exclusion can take various forms. The young woman who is intimidated by the atmosphere in a local bank lacks self-confidence to cope with an unfamiliar social environment and to interact with people she sees as belonging to a different social milieu from her own. The older person declaring, "I'm too thick" when offered a computer course also lacks self-confidence *and* has low self-esteem. When the Triangle project attempted to recruit a local researcher for the Gurnos/Galon Uchaf area, it was difficult to find anyone who thought they would be able to do the job. The undermining of confidence and self-esteem may have started at school or before but is continued in the type of face-to-face encounters described above. The problem appears to be wholly personal (psychological even), but it is, in a very Durkheimian sense, a *social* problem; the problem lies in the image of yourself that you see in the eyes of others. So the remedy lies, in part, in overcoming or re-evaluating others' perceptions of yourself and in demonstrating to yourself and others that you are a person capable of opening a bank account, using a computer or collecting information. We should not confuse this with building *social capital*, although, as we shall see, the two are intimately linked. The literature on social capital has been extensively reviewed (see Bourdieu, 1985; Coleman, 1998; Portes, 1998; ONS, 2001) and the intention is not to revisit this material here.

Social exclusion impinges on health. Being demeaned and demoralised (and denied access to services) may lead to loss of self-esteem and, while the direct links between self-esteem and health are not easy to demonstrate, it nevertheless appears to be the case that people under 25 with low self-esteem are more likely than others to show symptoms of depression, to be victimised and to have more difficulty forming and sustaining successful close relationships, and the girls are more likely to become pregnant as teenagers (Emler, 2001, p 59).

We might call issues of self-esteem and personal capacities problems of 'human capital' and follow Portes' succinct formulation of Bourdieu and Coleman:

> ... economic capital is in people's bank accounts and human capital is inside their heads, social capital inheres in the structure of their relationships. (1998, p 7)

It is the structure of relationships that determines the effectiveness of, say, Holway residents in negotiating with the housing department or bidding for funding for playing field improvements. There are two aspects to these capacities. First is the ability of Holway residents to work with one another, to agree their aims, marshal their evidence and agree who shall represent them. In doing this, they may have to overcome differences of interest (owner-occupiers versus council tenants, perhaps) and interpersonal conflicts (long-standing family feuds, for example). These conflicts were observed as being latent in nearly all attempts to organise activities and initiatives and sometimes manifest in undermining effective organisation. The capacity to sit on a committee – perhaps with gritted teeth – with people one does not like in order to achieve a specific objective is probably a capacity more commonly found in middle-class populations and institutions.

Reciprocity and trust are essential elements of social capital:

> The individual provides a service to others, or acts for the benefit of others at a personal cost, but in the general expectation that this kindness will be returned at some

> undefined time in the future in case of need. In a community
> where reciprocity is strong, people care for each other's
> interests. (Reno et al, cited in Onyx and Bullen, 2000)

It should be noted in passing that reciprocity is actually also one defining feature of a community. The word 'community' is used in policy literature when it may only be appropriate to refer to 'population'. The extent to which a community exists in a population is an empirical question that has to be explored, but this was done only obliquely in the SHARP research. The question was especially salient in the multicultural context of Cardiff Bay and was encountered by the Barefoot project and the south Riverside arm of the Triangle project.

Second, locally organised residents have to build the capacities that enable them to interact effectively with agencies outside the locality. These capacities may range from mobilising voters in order to exert pressure on a councillor to mounting a survey in order to produce data on local health or housing. It is important to note how far SHARP participants had to travel in this respect. A typical middle class-neighbourhood will often have sufficient numbers of articulate and self-confident residents to be able to organise a campaign, write letters to the press, ask questions in public and rebut points on their feet at meetings. The neighbourhood may also able to draw on the skills of resident professionals in planning, legal, educational, environmental and transport issues, for example. In working-class communities where there is a tradition of active trade unionism similar capacities may be present, but in areas like Holway and Pembrokeshire this has never been the case, or, in the Triangle project areas of Gurnos and Ystradgynlais the social foundations that supported such capacities have long drained away with unemployment and social exclusion. We might note in passing that successive government have actively undermined the trades union movement. In so doing, they have reduced the social capital of certain locations and destroyed an important channel through which individuals might have developed their personal capacities. With the decline of traditional industries, the close-knit networks of female kin and neighbours – conspicuous in early British community studies and very visible during the 1984-85 miners' strike – seem also to have declined.

What is necessary, therefore, is the development of two kinds of social capital, first, that needed to build local social cohesion and to enable local people to work together, and, second, that needed for local people to interact effectively beyond their immediate locality and possibly draw on the resources of outside agencies for their locality. These two forms of social capital have been described as 'bonding' and 'bridging'.

In Putnam's terms, bonding social capital enables you to 'get by', while bridging social capital enables you to 'get on' (Putnam, 2000).

The deprivation and social exclusion analyses (especially in the moral underclass version) posit a deficit model of the populations concerned. But in Pembrokeshire and on the Holway estate people spoke of the importance of good neighbours and how friendly and helpful local people could be. Furthermore, Oscar Lewis, in the passage cited above and elsewhere, demonstrated that bonding does not necessarily overcome deprivation and exclusion; it may actually reinforce them. Neighbourliness was strongly in evidence in Llanychaer in Pembrokeshire where long-lasting reciprocal bonds were formed between farming families who assisted one another with the essential and labour-intensive tasks that arose in the course of every farming year. But on the whole people in Pembrokeshire regretted the passing of neighbourliness. In south Riverside in Cardiff there is strong bonding within each of the numerous minority ethnic groups in the area, but less bridging to other groups, something that the Triangle and Barefoot projects attempted to build, particularly among minority ethnic women. We observed strong bonds on the Holway estate, for example, between small groups of young men. The effects of this are largely negative for the locality because the young men have a culture that is indifferent or hostile to education and stresses the kind of 'mucking around' that leads to antisocial behaviour; needless to say, this is not a culture that values gainful employment. The older bingo players also have social capital: they have a network of friends that extends beyond the estate to kin and former residents, they have a warm and sociable culture expressed in the weekly bingo sessions, they have relative economic security through their pensions and benefit entitlements, and they express satisfaction with the health and other public services they use. The 'connectedness' of older people was also noted by David Page in his study of three estates (Page, 2000, p 22). One consequence of this bonding is that the older people, often with occupational and domestic skills and valuable life experiences, do not need to make a contribution to the wider locality. They felt they had nothing to gain by joining with SHARP in the Holway estate, for example, but were worried that SHARP activities would impinge on their use of the community centre for bingo. Thus a potentially valuable local resource to be found in older people was not fully utilisable in the Holway project. It was also the case that older people felt especially threatened by the 'street' culture of the younger men, although younger people felt even less safe on the streets than their elders.

It should be noted, therefore, that strong bonds may have negative impacts. Furthermore, the proximity of supportive kin can make it harder to move away in pursuit of employment, whereas people with fewer local ties will find it easier to move away or adopt locally less conventional strategies – such as the young people who worked hard at school and the handful who went on to higher education. These considerations are sometimes summarised as the weakness of strong bonds and the strength of weak bonds. Certainly, some SHARP participants who were successful in gaining employment became much less active in community activities, both because of the demands of work and because they were able to distance themselves from the people who had not 'got on'. As is the case in many communities, including the Pembrokeshire SHARP locations and the Holway estate, people who got on tended to 'get out'. The role of family – both nuclear and extended – can therefore be an ambiguous one. The family is itself an element of social capital; it provides support for members and is able to transfer capacities and social skills to members. Families that break up either through failed relationships or by geographical mobility are less able to provide support and transmit elements of social capital. At the same time, the social capital found in the family may be just the kind of strong bond that prevents people getting on – especially if the skills it has to transmit are solely those of getting by and adapting to deprivation.

Partnership

'Partnership' has been a buzz word in British policy circles since the 1980s (but see Moore, 1997, pp 168-170). By the time SHARP was launched, it had become a central feature of policy innovation. Virtually no bid for project funding from local government or the voluntary sector could be entertained without firm evidence of partnership. In the competition for resources, 'paper' partnerships were not uncommon, but funders increasingly required evidence of effective partnership to be written into bids. This has had the effect of creating a financial incentive for both statutory and voluntary sector organisations. Some organisations nevertheless had non-financial incentives for partnership. The police, for example, appreciated that effective policing entailed working *with* the local population to address their needs. Groundwork and the Prince's Trust had not been able to establish any activities in the Flintshire/Denbighshire area and were therefore looking for an entrée of the kind that SHARP provided. Once established in the Holway project, Sure Start found that the take-up of its services for young mothers and their children was higher, because they were based in the locality and used local young women as helpers. Most conspicuously, the local authority needed to be able to initiate action on housing and the environment on the Holway estate; previous initiatives had been undermined by the frustration and hostility expressed in 'shouting matches'. All these agencies therefore had a need for partnership and the more effective the partnership proved to be, the more it created a bridge between local people and the agencies whose resources and services they wished to access. Partnership was an important feature of a number of projects (see Chapter Four) and as such comprised social capital of the 'bridging' kind for the population. Where partnership was less effective, opportunities for building social capital were absent. The creation of social capital through partnership was a two-way process as evidenced by interviews conducted in the Holway project. Their experience in Holway had enabled some voluntary sector partner agencies to operate more effectively in other locations, and it provided them with 'good practice' to take to these locations and a network of peers in potentially collaborating agencies. When professionals working in the voluntary sector said that SHARP had enabled them to meet people they would not otherwise have met, and that these were *useful* contacts, they were saying that their capacity to do their work had been enhanced and that *their* social capital had been increased.

Action research

It is debatable whether a project with research in the title was a good basis for action. Deprived populations and locations can have a long history of small projects and research which, because they lead nowhere, appear as a *substitute* for effective action. Researchers in Pembrokeshire, Cardiff Bay, the Triangle Project and the Holway all encountered such local histories.

Decades of purportedly benevolent research and regeneration activities are perceived to have made little contribution to the improvement of the social and economic conditions of these communities and, some might argue, have further stigmatised them (Carlisle et al, 2004, p 69). Minority ethnic communities perhaps suffer most from over-research and 'project-itis' and evidence from the Barefoot project suggests that local people believed this had generated a one-way flow of data about minorities without any tangible benefits for them. In the end, communities 'don't give a monkey's' about research – they just want to see action (Carlisle et al, 2004, p 73).

Yet the experience of Right 2 Respect and the Holway project is that 'look, think, act, review' is a valuable process that enables activities to be organised more effectively and a better case to be made for external support. But the appreciation of this needs to grow out of the experience of a project, and the benefits are not self-evident to most local people at the beginning of a project.

Working with people in the SHARP programme provided an opportunity to observe processes that are not trapped by surveys or hit-and-run focus group studies. Developing action research in this way, 'close up', for five years, must be almost unique for a government-funded project. The researchers worked especially 'close up' to the people who were the subjects of the research, so close that they became active participants in the projects and needed to maintain a critical and reflexive stance through which they were able to see themselves as part of the subject matter. This was especially the case for those researchers who were recruited from the local population that they were to be researching and who needed support in maintaining their twin roles of local researcher and local resident.

For any researcher working over a sustained period in one location, there is always a problem of confidentiality – the very richness of the material obtained makes much of it traceable to known individuals and, furthermore, in the daily life of research, one accumulates personal information that may not be directly relevant to the research. Long-term researchers also form friendships and acquire obligations and responsibilities to others in their locality. In the SHARP projects, the researchers' obligations to protect the identities of informants and others mean that much of the material gathered cannot be used. This is an acute problem for most locally recruited researchers who will have to live and work with the people and organisations in the locality after the research is finished, as one reported:

> Some things go on that you don't want to write about – you form friendships with people. But we're employed as researchers so we try to be an outsider. But your future's dependent on local relationships, so we can't be over-critical of other agencies. (Carlisle et al, 2004, p 75)

One extreme case was in the Barefoot project where the female researchers were highly visible and subject to continuous and critical male scrutiny. Perhaps each researcher now needs to write in some kind of fictional form in which they can argue out the issues raised in SHARP.

That working 'up close' has considerable benefits was expressed by one SHARP participant as follows:

> You can't really capture what a 15 year old girl is thinking about with a piece of paper with numbers on it. It may not seem a lot but I know that a girl who's taken part in nothing then starts taking part and going to places, as a girl who was quite apathetic or disinterested then gets an overall on and starts painting a room – they're changes you can't capture in numbers. (Carlisle et al, 2004, p 108)

A lack of trust was evident among some SHARP participants and this inhibited the development of the social capital that would have enabled local people to negotiate effectively with, for example, the local authority. Squabbles arose at meetings and escalated to an intensity that seemed entirely disproportionate to matters of slight disagreement. It was many months, in some cases years, before researchers discovered the history of interpersonal or family disputes that fuelled these conflicts. The disputes may have lasted for more than a generation, but they were a contemporary barrier to effective collective action and vivid demonstrations of ways in which 'the personal is political'. These encounters dramatically demonstrated the intersection of history and biography in small sections of the Welsh population.

The phrase the 'personal is political' has its origin in feminist thought and it expresses the view that our personal lives are in large measure politically delimited and determined so that in order to improve our personal relations we must address political structures. The Holway and other project sites reversed the order of this; in order to address political structures, people had to improve their personal relations. Over time it was possible to observe the growth of trust – or at least truce – through which individuals with long-standing grievances against one another came to work together for pragmatic ends. It is not known whether reconciliation and trust will develop further in the long run but the researchers would not have appreciated the extent of this issue without long-term, close involvement with the people in the projects.

From 'close up', SHARP researchers also observed women in the Holway project who were initially withdrawn and lacking self-confidence (some seldom leaving their houses) taking part in activities half way through the project and then beginning to organise them themselves. Some had even travelled to see similar initiatives in other locations. This progress took many months and was sometimes set back by personal conflicts or perceived slights; it entailed women being invited to join in, being taken along and encouraged either by project workers or by other local women who had more confidence. Others needed help with literacy in order to pass the driving test, or to help their children when they started school. All the projects reported progress by very small steps. Having or regaining the confidence to make a telephone call to a local authority office may not seem much to an outsider, but in personal terms this could be a very big step for a person who had experienced rejection with contempt by others. In the second half of the project, many Holway residents said that five years ago they could not have imaged themselves today – undertaking work in the community, using the internet, having a driving licence or a European Computer Driving Licence, or gaining qualifications in youth work or childcare. In all projects, a number of local people were encouraged and supported in acquiring formal (often entry-level) qualifications as a possible means of entry to the labour market. The young women who had learnt desk-top publishing and were taking a journalism course in the Right 2 Respect project had experienced a transformation of their image of themselves, were becoming an asset to their peers and locality and were acquiring skills and self-confidence that would be valuable in seeking employment. They were also creating a vehicle for the circulation of information of value to the local population, as were the residents who produced the Holway newsletter – individual skills thus became community assets and instruments of local empowerment. Human capital becomes social capital. The Holway women who took floristry courses and an introduction to business through Stepping Out to Independence later discussed setting up a local floristry business. Although this had not materialised by the end of the SHARP project, the women had gained the experience of planning a business venture together. Their collective capacity remains in the locality. A woman in the Triangle project reported:

> I'm living proof that it's possible to overcome even the most difficult experiences in life, which do happen. The way I feel about myself now is that I can feel positive towards life once again, and I feel this happened through me being able to access the support that was there. (Triangle, 2000, p 18)

The women who trained as lifeguards in Cardiff will be employed at local swimming pools to enable other women to swim at women-only sessions. As well as providing others with an opportunity to improve their health and sense of wellbeing through swimming, these women will set an example to those who feel isolated in the community by demonstrating improved self-confidence and an ability to gain part-time employment. They will also set an example of self-improvement to their own children and other girls in the minority community. Beyond this, human and social capital can become economic capital when acquired skills and enhanced self-confidence put money in the bank through employment.

In both the BeWEHL (Bettws Women's Education, Health and Lifestyle) and Holway projects, participants reported a decline in the use of anti-depressants. This is of particular interest because it is an indicator of improving health that is not likely to be picked up in any analysis by GPs or the local health authority and furthermore no survey of the use of prescription drugs would have been feasible in the SHARP areas. In the Barefoot project, a woman overcame her depression by participating in project events; she began to enjoy herself, her talents were acknowledged by others and she felt valued as a person again. By the end of the project, she had established a small business. For one person, this was long journey within the lifetime of the SHARP project. Perhaps, like a participant in another of the projects, she could have said:

> The project has helped me remember who I am – it helped me to find myself again. (Carlisle et al, 2004, p 118)

The growth of self-esteem and self-confidence, and the acquisition of knowledge and skills by individuals is the development of human capital, viewed 'close up', and it is intimately linked to social capital because it is in their relations with others in the locality that individuals' self-esteem, self-confidence and – therefore – human capital grows. What they see in the eyes of others is an enhanced image of themselves as someone who has a contribution to make. The resulting gain in confidence enables them to extend their capabilities further. There is 'positive feedback' and the researchers were able to observe this in their daily encounters. Self-esteem and social capital rise in a virtuous circle. People who have made the progression are able to help others make the same progression – they are an asset that is more or less available to the locality, as in the case of the lifeguards in Cardiff and the young women in Wrexham. There is no boundary between human and social capital – they are reciprocal and complementary. Thus we see that individuals have overcome labour market exclusion by finding employment through acquiring driving licenses, knowledge of floristry and the ability to swim, for example. Others have directly overcome market exclusion by setting up food cooperatives that bring fresh food to their community at affordable prices. Others are laying the foundation either for entering the labour market, by improving their literacy or computer skills, or acquiring the self-esteem and knowledge that will enable them better to equip their children to thrive, by helping them with their school work and setting a good example as self-confident parents. None of this can happen until people 'feel better about themselves' and when it does, they feel even better about themselves.

These successes, closely observed at a local and personal level, do not overcome the causes of inequality and exclusion. SHARP enabled people to access available resources ranging from grants for CCTV to support from the Prince's Trust and Groundwork. Personnel from the voluntary sector, local government development workers and university staff then became links to wider political structures. In the case of Holway, the encouragement of a 'look, think, act, review' culture enabled residents to make organised and informed approaches to the county council for assistance with serious housing problems. That local people were now being listened to was in itself a source of pride and perhaps created a sense of empowerment. One striking example of effective partnership was that between the Holway Tenants' and Residents' Association, the local authority, the police and a university researcher in dealing with a private landlord who was reluctant to address the problem of unruly tenants who were disrupting the life of a street. No one partner would have succeeded alone. At the end of the SHARP programme, the issue for many if not most of those who have become involved in all seven projects was to sustain partnerships that make this kind of action possible after the projects have finished. None of the SHARP project communities or participants will become, or become part of, an economically, socially and politically self-sustaining 'community'. Part of the continuing capacity of the participants in the Triangle, Barefoot, Pembrokeshire and Holway projects will be their ability to draw down expertise and resources through the networks established during the project. The social capital of SHARP participants is not in their bank balances or their heads, but 'inheres in the structure of their relationships' within their locality and with outside agencies.

Through Levitas's redistributive discourse on social exclusion, we see that SHARP has enjoyed its successes *within* an economic and political system that is deeply unequal and that SHARP was not intended to address. It is as if the objective of inclusion policies is

> ... merely to move [the excluded] across a boundary, leaving underlying structural divisions largely undisturbed. (Goodin, cited in Lister, 2004, p 81)

We have also seen the limits of what partnership can achieve: SHARP was a health project yet the institutions of the National Health Service were conspicuous by their absence right across the programme. Unlike, say, Sure Start or the Prince's Trust, agencies of the NHS had no *interest* in SHARP and therefore no incentive to build partnerships. Local GPs, for example, would not see the results of improved diet and raised levels of exercise among their patients for a decade or two, or until after their retirement. There was no obvious payback for joining in partnership and therefore little incentive to implement the vision set out in Chapter 3 of *Improving Health in Wales* (National Assembly for Wales, 2001). The hospital trusts were inextricably engaged with the issue of waiting lists to the exclusion of nearly all other matters. There would be no immediate or tangible benefit to them to become SHARP partners – even though in 20 years' time SHARP may have reduced the incidence of emergency admissions for coronary heart disease from the local populations.

The government's crime and disorder agenda did give the police a direct interest in partnership with local people on the Holway estate. The residents for their part had a number of issues relating to traffic, crime and antisocial behaviour that they wished to see addressed urgently. Here there was a convergence of interests with an effective partnership emerging out of some conflictful early engagements between the eventual partners. All the parties had a direct interest in the success of the partnership; the partnership drew in substantial external resources and enabled the police to focus on issues of local concern – which happily coincided with national crime and disorder objectives. No amount of personal empowerment or local social capital would have been sufficient to achieve these ends without the framework created by national policing priorities. The Holway experience became a resource for the police and for other communities. That the police emerged as one of the most progressive forces in the Holway project may in some part be due to the good intentions of the people involved, but it was mainly due to the coincidence of *interests* that enabled national and region resources to be 'bent' to the interests of local people

Residents in Wales, as in England, are beset by the problems created by the reduction of resources for the local services they need, which special initiatives and projects like SHARP cannot mask (Page, 2000, pp 53-65). Holway residents could not take any action to overcome either the lack of resources for public housing or the chronic mismanagement of the Flintshire housing maintenance and repairs department. Thus in spite of their orderly approaches to the local authority – who listened to them carefully – no effective action was taken on housing, which was, with crime and disorder, the single issue that most concerned local residents throughout the project. Yet poor housing was possibly having the largest single detrimental effect on the physical and mental health of estate residents, something recognised by the Welsh Assembly Government in a number of documents, including the 2002 *Well Being in Wales* consultation document (§7.5).

Conclusion

What was special about the people of the SHARP project? None of the populations involved was homogeneous; there were people in and out of work, retired people, teenage women at school hoping to go to college or university, and others with babies. Some residents in the SHARP estates were long established and others were newcomers. Some young residents came from secure family backgrounds and received continuing support from them, while others had come out of care and lacked domestic skills and supportive relationships. There were some residents for whom chronic ill health, either physical or mental, made their future prospects very poor. There were few people who did not share some or all of the aspirations widely held across society: a decent home, healthy children, a peaceful life, holidays, and nice clothes. They enjoyed popular TV programmes; 'Coronation Street' or 'Bad Girls' could depopulate a meeting if the latter ran over the time of the programme. Some of the older people were content: they could look back on a working life with some pride, they enjoyed a wide circle of kin and friends, they were economically secure, and although not affluent, they owned their own homes or rented higher-quality council houses. They, like some of those in work, were, as Page discovered in his research (Page, 2000), 'connected', whereas those not in work were less connected with people, agencies and activities outside their immediate locality. To this extent, there was nothing special about Holway residents or any of the people living in the SHARP project areas.

Yet SHARP people *were* different, mainly by virtue of the degree to which they experienced deprivation and exclusion. By definition, SHARP locations could not be populated by affluent people. This meant that many of the project participants did not enjoy the holidays advertised on television, very few had a new car and old 'bangers' were common on the streets. Few of the core populations had well-paid work and many did not have any work at all. SHARP participants did not enjoy high levels of consumption of public services, the availability and quality of public services, notably housing, has declined in recent decades and low incomes are supported by benefits administered with increasingly complicated entitlement rules and harsh regulation (Jones and Novak, 1999). SHARP participants tended to be part of the population that these changes targeted. The people who were seen by the Welsh Assembly Government as being at the heart of the SHARP project knew where they stood in society and how they were regarded by other citizens and by the state. They 'knew their place'.

Not being able to share in the patterns of consumption that are represented and celebrated on television is, no doubt, a form of *relative* deprivation, but it is one shared with the majority of the population that does not have a new car or a foreign holiday every year. However, sections of the SHARP populations also endure degrees of absolute poverty, lacking essential items, in some cases making do with older clothes and shoes, and lacking well-equipped kitchens. For a significant minority, indebtedness is an additional problem; how to balance outstanding bills can become a major preoccupation, especially for younger and less experienced men and women. While there are adequate transport services in the more urban SHARP areas, people are nevertheless isolated by their deprivation – they shop only for the basics. Those who could afford nice furnishings or other goods for their homes would be wasting their money if they lived in the concrete houses in the Holway or similarly cold and damp houses or private rented dwellings elsewhere. The impersonal forces of the market and the welfare state therefore exclude people from realising their aspirations. For people below retirement age, the lack of employment, or the lack of an employed person bringing an income into the household, is a serious cause of deprivation.

Women bear the brunt of the stressful tasks of managing a household and its debts. If they have a non-working or dependent partner, especially one with an alcohol or drug problem, they are subject to even greater stress. Yet women felt relatively defenceless, vulnerable *and* shamed by not 'having a man'. It is not surprising, therefore, that the use of anti-depressants was quite widespread among women. The incidence of smoking was also high among SHARP populations. Long exposure to reduced circumstances undermine hope and lead to lower aspirations and eventually to a devaluation of self – it is easy to feel a failure, to blame oneself, to see oneself as inadequate. This is especially the case where this sense of inadequacy is reinforced through contacts with others and the stigma attached to the place you live and to people like you by the local press, by politicians and the national media. It is not hard to see why people become addicted to prescription drugs or graduate from them to illicit drugs, alcohol and tobacco. In addressing these problems, SHARP's apparently small achievements constitute significant and substantial successes.

In the conditions described, young people have little to aspire for, there are no jobs and parents are neither striving nor achieving in the outside world – they may not even be providing regular meals. There are no effective role models. There are alternative role models to be found in the drug dealers who seem never to be short of cash; there is the life of the street with everything from breaking windows to stealing cars to provide a 'buzz'. In such circumstances, young people have little or no interest in schoolwork and drop out into an alternative, truant, culture. Their parents either have no means of controlling this behaviour or share the view that there is little to be gained from schooling. In such a context, the establishment of a homework club is a significant achievement.

The importance of work cannot be underestimated, but for many the pursuit of low-paid work has too many hazards, notably negotiating oneself off and on benefits, with the inevitable severe loss of income in the transition from work to unemployment. To be better off in work, people on benefits need to earn at least £200 to £250 a week, and such jobs are hard to come by. In the late 1990s, a group in the Holway project was discussing the salary advertised for a local authority job. At £12,000 a year, it was not 'a Mickey Mouse job', they said. The job and the income (about half the median income for England and Wales) were beyond their aspirations. Projects like SHARP cannot change the occupation structure or wages policies but they can help people negotiate economic hazards.

Making benefit allocation harsher will not get people back into work. Furthermore, the thrust towards paid employment as the solution to social exclusion devalues caring and family work, including raising children, and also undervalues the importance of voluntary activities undertaken in the locality. As well as being beneficial in themselves, these activities have monetary value for the state that largely remains unrecognised. But even if jobs were available, the people in these locations lack appropriate skills and work experience. To acquire skills, they may need first to improve their literacy and numeracy. The lack of these basic skills can itself be a source of low self-esteem and self-confidence, making entry or re-entry to the labour market a daunting or seemingly impossible prospect. So, for the majority of those who would be called 'excluded', the experience in SHARP suggests that a single leap from exclusion to employment is not possible (even if it is desirable).

Direct approaches to what people perceive to be their inadequacies will reinforce a sense of inadequacy and be rebuffed. Learning to help children with schoolwork and being rewarded with driving lessons for being useful in the locality enabled people to gain skills and self-confidence without any loss of self-esteem. Doing these things with others builds up networks of peers who can share the frustration and fun of improving their spelling. Then it is an easier step to undertake craft activities and perhaps contribute to a food cooperative. Young men with no employment experience or 'discouraged unemployed' can help with digging or painting on a community project, 'for a laugh' perhaps, maybe to enjoy the sunshine and the female company. They may win praise for their efforts and perhaps meet voluntary sector participants who tell them how they might develop this first step towards employment *and* offer help in making a telephone call or providing a lift to an interview. These beginnings are very small and they are easily set back, by anything from a disparaging comment to a hangover. The beginnings need continual support from the public and voluntary sector, not the professional support of statutory agencies, but the friendship and encouragement of someone who listens and never mocks your efforts.

Out of these small-scale experiences grow the collective capacities – the 'social capital', first 'bonding', then 'bridging'. This capital too is easily destroyed, especially when the hopes raised by a project like SHARP are not realised. Another failed or unsustainable project could move a locality – and its people – backwards.

References

Barry, D. (2002) *A Bloody Good Friday*, London: Cape.

Boreham, R., Stafford, M. and Taylor, R. (2000) *Health Survey for England 2000: Social Capital and Health*, London: The Stationery Office.

Bourdieu, P. (1985) 'The forms of capital', in G.G. Richardson (ed) *Handbook of Theory and Research for the Sociology of Education*, New York, NY: Greenwood.

Brewer, M., Browne, J. and Sutherland, H. (2006a) *Micro-simulating Child Poverty in 2010 and 2020*, London: Institute for Fiscal Studies.

Brewer, M., Goodman, A. and Leicester, A. (2006b) *Household Spending in Britain: What can it Teach us about Poverty?*, London: Institute of Fiscal Studies.

Carlisle, S., Cropper, S., Beech, R. and Little, R. (2004, unpublished) 'SHARP Overarching Evaluation Team Phase 2 Report', Keele: Keele University.

Coleman, J.S. (1988) 'Social capital and the creation of human capital', *American Journal of Sociology, Supplement: Organisations and Institutions: Sociological and Economic Approaches to the Analysis of Social Structure*, vol 94, S95–S120.

Emler, N. (2001) *Self-esteem: The Costs and Causes of Low Self-worth*, York: Joseph Rowntree Foundation.

Gordon, D. (2005) 'Can we make poverty history?', *Radical Statistics*, no 89, pp 13–28.

Graham, H. (2004) 'Tackling health inequalities in England: remedying health disadvantages, narrowing gaps or reducing health gradients', *Journal of Social Policy*, no 33, pp 115–31.

Gravelle, H. (1998) 'How much of the relation between population mortality and unequal distribution of income is a statistical artefact?', *British Medical Journal*, no 316, pp 382–5.

Griffiths, N. (2001) *Grits*, London: Vintage.

Jones, C. and Novak, T. (1999) *Poverty, Welfare and the Disciplinary State*, London and New York, NY: Routledge.

Judge, K. (1995) 'Income distribution and life expectancy: a critical appraisal', *British Medical Journal*, no 311, pp 1282–5.

Levitas, R. (1996) 'The concept of social exclusion and the new Durkheimian hegemony', *Critical Social Policy*, no 46, pp 5–20.

Levitas, R. (2000) 'What is social exclusion', in D. Gordon and P. Townsend (eds) *Breadline Europe: The Measurement of Poverty*, Bristol: The Policy Press.

Levitas, R. (2006) 'The concept and measurement of social exclusion', in C. Pantazis, D. Gordon and R. Levitas (eds) *Poverty and Social Exclusion in Britain: The Millennium Survey,* Bristol: The Policy Press.

Lewis, O. (1968) *A Study of Slum Culture: Backgrounds for La Vida*, New York, NY: Random House.

Lister, R. (2004) *Poverty*, Cambridge: Polity Press.

Moore, R. (1997) 'Poverty and partnership in the Third European Poverty Programme: the Liverpool case', in N. Jewson and S. MacGregor (eds) *Transforming Cities*, London: Routledge, pp 166–78.

Moore, R. (2001) 'Rediscovering the underclass', in R. Burgess and A. Murcott (eds) *Developments in Sociology*, Harlow: Prentice Hall.

National Assembly for Wales (2001a) *Improving Health in Wales: A Plan for the NHS with its Partners*, Cardiff: National Assembly for Wales.

National Assembly for Wales (2001b) *Promoting Health and Well Being: Implementing the National Health Strategy*, Cardiff: National Assembly for Wales.

Onyx, J. and Bullen, P. (2000) 'Measuring social capital in five communities', *Journal of Applied Behavioural Science*, vol 36, no 1, pp 23-42.

Page, D. (2000) *Communities in the Balance*, York: Joseph Rowntree Foundation.

Pantazis, C., Gordon, D. and Levitas, R. (eds) (2006) *Poverty and Social Exclusion in Britain: The Millennium Survey*, Bristol: The Policy Press.

Pevalin, D.J. and Rose, D. (2003) *Social Capital for Health: Investigating the Links between Social Capital and Health using the British Household Panel Survey*, London: Health Development Agency.

Piachaud, D. and Sutherland, H. (2000) *How Effective is the British Government's Attempt to Reduce Child Poverty?*, London: Centre for Analysis of Social Exclusion, London School of Economics and Political Science.

Portes, A. (1998) 'Social capital: its origins and application in modern sociology', *Annual Review of Sociology*, vol 24, pp 1-24.

Putnam, R. (2000) *Bowling Alone: The Collapse and Revival of American Community*, New York: Simon and Schuster.

SEU (Social Exclusion Unit) (1997) *Social Exclusion Unit: Purpose, Work Priorities and Working Methods*, London: SEU.

SEU (2001) *Social Capital: A Review of the Literature*, London: Office for National Statistics.

Sutherland, H. (2000) *The British Government's Attempt to Reduce Child Poverty: A Budget 2000 Postscript*, Microsimulation Unit Research Note 36, Colchester: Microsimulation Unit.

Sutherland, H., Sefton, T. and Piachaud, D. (2003) *Poverty in Britain: The Impact of Government Policy since 1997*, York: Joseph Rowntree Foundation.

Townsend, P. (1979) *Poverty in the United Kingdom*, London: Penguin.

Triangle (2005) *Phase 2 Report*, Cardiff: School of Social Sciences, University of Wales.

Welsh Assembly Government (2002) *Well Being in Wales: Consultation Document*, Cardiff: Welsh Assembly Government.

Welsh Assembly Government (2005) *Wales: A Vibrant Economy: The Welsh Assembly Government's Strategic Framework for Economic Development*, Cardiff: Welsh Assembly Government.

Welsh Office (1998) *Better Health – Better Wales*, Cm 3922, Cardiff: The Stationery Office.

Wilkinson, R.G. (1995) 'A reply to Ken Judge: mistaken criticisms ignore overwhelming evidence', *British Medical Journal*, vol 311, pp 1285-7.

NINE

Beyond the experimenting society

Gareth Williams, Steve Cropper, Alison Porter and Helen Snooks

Introduction

The poor health in some of Wales' more deprived communities could make the Sustainable Health Action Research Programme (SHARP) seem less like a bold experiment and more like a very inadequate sticking plaster on a deep and bloody wound. Nonetheless, to fund seven action research projects of the kind discussed in this book over a relatively long time period, as part of the wider programme of policy development, signalled a genuine commitment to a radical approach to health improvement for Wales. As Robert Moore indicated in Chapter Eight, the programme of community-based, public health-orientated action research to address health problems in disadvantaged communities was captured most clearly and forcefully in the Welsh context in *Better Health – Better Wales* (Welsh Office, 1998), a White Paper in which a distinctively Welsh agenda for health was set out for the first time. Within this agenda, SHARP emerged as a clear, but unelaborated, commitment to developing a health improvement strategy that recognised the social determinants of health and did more than reiterate the need for individual behaviour change.

It is easy when confronted by the immediate problems of poor health to put aside everything that is known about the wider determinants of health and the need for 'upstream' solutions. This is partly because of the popular and media pressure to deal with health (or sickness) services, waiting times and the availability of new treatments. However, it is also because, for all our considerable knowledge of the determinants of health, the links between socioeconomic position and mortality and the patterns of limiting long-term illness, evidence on specific interventions to address these problems is less easily identified, less robust, or so focused on one particular issue that the important wider context disappears from view. While there are growing numbers of specific interventions to address, say, tobacco use and diet among children and young people, broader community-based initiatives have been less easy to implement and test. They are 'wicked problems', as Steve Cropper and Mark Goodwin note in Chapter Two, for which simple evidence-based prescriptions are not readily available – interventions are about institutional and institutionalised change as much as the adoption or establishment of a service.

In principle, the lack of a strong body of evidence for community-level interventions militated against such a commitment. In England, the Health Action Zones were formed in the context of a wider programme of action that drew on measures of need and on the general principle of area-based intervention. SHARP was unusual in being defined primarily as a programme of research rather than as an initiative and, in the context of the vested interests that normally dictate any kind of spending on health-related activities, the programme represented a considerable achievement for a new health and social services minister, in an infant Assembly, supported by a civil service still coming to grips with the enlarged responsibilities brought by devolution. It was specifically community- rather than area-focused and included communities of identity as well as communities of place in the seven projects. It represented an attempt creatively to fuse three principles – responsiveness to community, partnership among agencies and organisations, and action research – in order to provoke innovation in both aspects of policy to which Chapter Two refers: the substance of policy, on the one hand, and the process or procedures of policy making on the other.

As indicated elsewhere in this book, much of the evidence on social determinants of health indicates that the most important determinants are nothing to do with the institutional domain of health at all. They are concerned with economic development, education, housing, regeneration and justice, and so the widest set of social institutions – public services including the police, schools, voluntary organisations, housing and transport providers, employment services and employers – are implicated in the call to action that policy on health inequalities represents. Chapter Three discussed the relatively few initiatives in the UK and elsewhere that have attempted to install large-scale programmes and policies while keeping a strong community focus. Although it may not constitute a 'large-scale experiment', SHARP is another example of this kind of work. It is a programme that has sought, systematically, to add to understanding both of the character of health inequalities and of the possibilities for taking intelligent local action to address those inequalities.

Social exclusion and inclusion

The processes of inquiry initiated by SHARP have been focused on the development of conceptions of inequalities that emerge from the search for 'intelligent action'. In this sense, its significance is perhaps to be found in the consistent and sustained engagement in an active process of inquiry and of development *with* communities. This was a mutual and reciprocal process, one that understands these communities as embedded in history, society and culture. In Chapter Three, Porter and Roberts drew on Levitas' analysis of three discourses of social exclusion and the forms of action they suggest. From its initiation, SHARP was defined most clearly in terms of what Levitas (1998) calls the social inclusion discourse (SID), for which interventions aimed at reducing social isolation and low self-esteem through building community activity and social capital reflect the way exclusion is constructed. The brief to SHARP projects and to the overarching evaluation, for example, specified the development of social capital as an area for inquiry within the programme. Moore's commentary on the outcomes of SHARP in Chapter Eight also reflects the dominant conception of community wellbeing and health inequalities in terms of SID. And it is this sense of exclusion as much as the lack of material resources that members of communities saw as the core of their problems. Moore's appraisal of the difference made by SHARP gives greatest significance to interventions aimed at reducing social isolation and low self-esteem through building community activity and social capital.

The concept of social capital is often used as a construct to be operationalised and measured, and at other times it is employed more as a metaphor, helping to orientate researchers and activists towards the particular kinds of action and practice in which they are involved. It is in this second 'generative' sense that social capital has been most relevant in the work of SHARP, where working out what the implications of ideas could be for concrete action in the specific community settings has been a central task. In many of the projects, social capital has not been the metaphor with greatest generative force; rather, the idea of 'community' has served as the primary generative mechanism, taken together with those of 'health' and the 'wider determinants of health'. Nevertheless, as Chapter Five suggests, the diagnoses of community and the manner of thinking about 'what to do' are thoroughly infused with social capital – networking, brokerage across separate parts of communities, small-scale exchange, unconditional 'giving', work to develop trust, and work on self-regard, respect and mutual regard have all been central to SHARP action and to the research activity that has gone with the action in different ways.

The question of whether it is possible to create and support social capital in communities where opportunities are few and resilience is low is an important one (Cropper, 2002). SHARP's consistent focus has been on creating opportunities for collectively meaningful interaction. While interventions to address individual lifestyle factors were certainly a part of projects' work, these were understood socially. Activities that promoted physical activity or that focused on nutrition were also seen fundamentally as points around which social relations would form, both in the making of the activities and through the acts of participation. They were also seen as resources through which communities could regain a sense of focus, resourcefulness, achievement and pride.

Although social capital has tended to be discussed as a property of civil society (or community), sometimes referred to as bonding and bridging social capital within and across communities (Woolcock, 2001), many of the SHARP projects illustrate additionally the profound importance of what Woolcock and others characterise as 'linking' social capital, focusing our attention on relations between communities and the agencies that have service responsibilities. Others, too, (for example, Lowndes and Wilson, 2001; Pickin et al, 2002) have argued that links between communities and their local public organisations are the crucial component of this collective resource; and, further, that social capital formation is strongly shaped by the way local democratic and public service organisations have structured opportunities for public involvement.

As Cornwall's (2007) study in south Wales has shown, where 'bonding' social capital is strong because of shared social and economic adversity, it is sometimes very difficult to get members of neighbouring communities to talk to each other without shouting, or to get professionals in local agencies to respond to community mobilisation with anything approaching common decency and respect. It is significant, then, that the outcomes Moore cites in Chapter Eight include re-establishment of service relations and dialogue between communities and those agencies, where previously these had broken down, and the difficulties of reliance on long-established systems of representation. Such work to develop social capital has been pursued with both 'place-based' communities (such as Moore's involvement with the geographically tight Holway community, and the Triangle project's work, particularly in Merthyr Tydfil) and with communities of identity – Goodwin and Armstong-Esther (2004) report on social capital development among children and young people through HYPP (Health of Young People in Powys project).

In their assessment of what we now know about 'using evidence' in policy and practice to inform public services, Nutley and colleagues (2007) make three key arguments. First, they ask whether processes of learning and reciprocal influence around evidence or research emerge naturally among dynamic networks of actors or whether 'they can be created, encouraged, or stimulated by more deliberative action ..., how ... and by whom' (p 262). Second, they argue that the context in which policy is made is important in understanding the use of research in policy making and practice but, as yet, the connections are poorly understood. Third, they enlarge the very notion of using evidence to include both the widest set of forms of knowledge and the processes through which evidence is formed; and they note that this occurs when policy processes are 'opened up' to new voices, new forms of evidence and deliberative practices, representing a democratisation of policy. If policy is indeed made as much as implemented at local level, the knowledge used, and that emerging, may be less immediately tangible and appear less tidy than that representing the results of science and its methods. A shift away from an understanding of the use of evidence as purely instrumental (that is, 'facts' directly informing a decision) towards one that emphasises other mechanisms and outcomes (enriched social practice and dialogue, building social and political connections within policy communities, and indeed policy critique) is an important potential development in evidence-based policy.

Working from the bottom up

Although by no means unique in this regard, Wales has a long and honourable history of religious and secular organisations in the community and the workplace trying to develop forms of organisation and mutual aid in communities, often in situations of considerable opposition and struggle (Jones, 1982; Francis and Smith, 1998; Pope, 1998). These organisations provided resources in times of need, ideologies with which to handle the uncertainties of everyday life, education – both formal education in reading and writing and the informal development of administrative, public-speaking and debating skills – and healthcare. The medical aid societies, such as the Tredegar Medical Aid Society where Aneurin Bevan developed his skills as a health service administrator, were owned and controlled by their subscribers, and provided basic healthcare in times of medical need. Similarly, the south Wales coal miners' representatives engaged in highly sophisticated argument and debate with scientific experts of different kinds in pushing their claims for compensation for industrial diseases and injuries (Bloor, 2000). These kinds of development within working-class communities, driven very often by home-grown intellectuals, represented both an embryonic welfare state and a set of processes through which people became involved and developed skills in what we might nowadays refer to as the 'governance' of communities (see Smith (1993) for a lively discussion of the historical context of south Wales). While it would be excessively romantic to draw too direct a connection from these multiple histories in Wales to modern developments, these are clearly part of the cultural self-regard that can inform responses to contemporary developments. One implication for policy making is suggested: policy may have its origins in local practices, innovations and critiques of orthodoxy, but these require strong forms of local organisation. Communities and groups that are excluded and have little in the way of resources and support will also have limited capacity to contribute: yet, it is most important that they organise to make representations and that their voice is heard.

There have been some bold experiments elsewhere in the world in the past to bring together local communities, health and local authorities, and experts of different kinds. One well-known example is the 'poverty programme' launched, as Harrington (1971) recalls, as part of Lyndon Johnson's vision of the Great Society and his 'unconditional War on Poverty' in the US in the 1960s. As with SHARP, this involved a relatively small number of projects, funded by different means, representing what was at the time regarded as '… the most imaginative and ambitious attempt to manipulate deliberate social change' (xvii) (see also Gorman, 1995). While concentrating initially on the problem of poverty, '… it arose less from moral indignation at injustice than from a sense of breakdown in the institutions which should be diffusing opportunities for all' (Marris and Rein, 1974, p 23).

In their analysis of the process of reform, Marris and Rein argue that any reform 'faces three crucial tasks': recruiting a *coalition of power*; respecting the *democratic tradition*; and being *demonstrably rational* (1974, p 29). Translated into the language of our own time and place, we might say that any new policy or programme dealing with poverty, health inequalities or neighbourhood renewal should be based on a *stakeholder partnership*, facilitate *community engagement* and be *evidence-based*. For those who worry about how we can best measure the outcome of such policies or programmes – Are people better off? Has health improved? Is the neighbourhood more friendly and cohesive? – Marris and Rein make an important point in the preface to the second edition of their book. They state:

> We have also added a further chapter on community action as an attempt to revitalize the processes of democratic government, for it is in this sense – rather than as a means of relieving poverty – that we think it has the most lasting importance. (Marris and Rein, 1974, p 9)

Wales and the wider UK in the early 21st century offer very different economic, political and policy environments from those prevailing in the late 20th-century US, and for that reason any lessons from the past have to be interpreted and adapted to current conditions. However, without understanding the history of previous attempts to involve communities in change, it is all too easy to lose any analytical perspective on exactly what it is that such community-based projects do. The very concept of 'community' is so agreeable, so loveable to almost everyone, that it is easy to lose sight of the radical and challenging nature of programmes such as SHARP.

The importance of demonstrable rationality

What, then, can we learn from past efforts if the context in which projects take place has changed considerably? First, the question of the purpose of such programmes, what they can conceivably set out to do and how we should approach their assessment, is crucial. In Chapter Two, Steve Cropper and Mark Goodwin note Graham's argument that the first step in understanding what is to be done about health inequalities is to develop greater clarity in our goals, a clarity that is missing from many government documents.

Exworthy and Powell (2000) and Exworthy and colleagues (2002) have recorded the lack of agreement about, and shared commitment to, tackling health inequalities at local level in the UK. This may be justified in the face of equivocal evidence and weak force of instruction about what to do. However, there is evidence that organisational factors also militate against the development of progress through joint work. Exworthy and Powell's (2000) survey indicates that the conditions for effective partnerships are lacking, but that investment in a further locale for social capital (now termed 'organisational social capital' (Nahapiet and Ghoshal, 1998; Adler and Kwon, 2002) has helped to overcome inertia. A substantial literature on partnership and interagency working emphasises that personal connections and a framework mandate that sets direction but leaves the detail to be resolved are crucial resources if risks are to be taken, and learning and trust developed (Bardach, 1998; Sullivan and Skelcher, 2002; Huxham and Vangen, 2005).

In the past, tough, top-down, bureaucratic evaluation criteria have inevitably found the loose, bottom-up approach to community-based action research deficient and difficult to act on (Dennett et al, 1982). Marris and Rein's choice of the phrase 'demonstrably rational' (see also Jasanoff, 2007) is helpful in this regard, providing a much richer and more powerful framework for how we should approach the development, implementation and evaluation of such programmes than the eviscerated concept of 'evidence-based'. While the latter ties us down to rather limited notions of generalised evidence and conclusiveness, the former implies a looser, more multifaceted and potentially more contextually aware approach to assessing the success of what we do: whether it works and whether it matters if it works or not. As Chapter Two argues, the current emphasis on 'evidence-based policy' is really only relevant to certain kinds of simple, quite well-defined policy problems. By itself it is an insufficient approach to the problem of health inequalities with its uncertainties in both goals and the means to attain them. Where there are uncertainties or ambiguities in both means and ends, as with the wicked problem of health inequalities, we will probably be engaged in a mixture of policy learning and muddling through, rather than simply applying evidence to policy (see also Nutley et al, 2007).

The question of the significance of policy and social action and to whom is important in the context of the point made by Marris and Rein quoted above. While many researchers and policy makers would dearly love to stop crime, make people happy, abolish ill health and be able to evaluate how we have done so, demonstrable rationality encourages us to think of the success of programmes such as SHARP or Communities First in a more rounded way, and to look at them from a number of different points of view. If governments were able to think in terms of the demonstrably rational, it would make the interfaces between the design, implementation and evaluation of policy richer places for deliberation and governance.

The concept of demonstrable rationality is even more important in the context of the two other crucial tasks referred to by Marris and Rein. Although when stated in the abstract they seem self-evidently to be desirable ends, there are those who might question whether we would wish to eliminate poverty or abolish ill health at all costs. We could imagine a totally managed and controlled environment in which poverty and ill health had disappeared, but in which democratic traditions and processes had also disappeared, and there were no coalitions of power because power resides in one governing body. It is not our intention to pursue this exercise in political philosophy here, but simply to remind ourselves that controlled and tested experiments in living have their limits in the contexts of everyday civil society; contexts where we are also concerned with retaining democratic processes, and recognising the freedoms, powers and entitlements of different groups. So long as there remain opportunities for 'popular voice', competing values or uncertainty about 'ends' will remain a source of constraint in policy making, as values become translated into practical measures. Values also infuse the definition and choice of the means to improve wellbeing. In health policy, a range of types of measure is now conventionally defined in terms of the locus of responsibility for change – this defines the types of service that then follow. Two points on the spectrum have tended to dominate. In the health field, the whole of the 1980s and much of the 1990s saw conflict between what were entrenched positions on the state's responsibility for health. The strategy for health improvement articulated by the then Conservative government was almost wholly to do with individual behaviour, and the response from critics was that it was all to do with structure (Williams, 2006).

It is dispiriting to see the way in which governments can drift so easily back into a limited vision of health policy that emphasises hospital waiting times on the one hand and individual behaviour change on the other. Both strands of policy are easy to sell, for politicians on the stump and for the media. The overwhelming evidence is that health policy dominated by these twin foci will do little to improve the health of the majority of the population and will widen the gap that already exists between rich and poor people, between people with access to resources and assets and people with access to few of these, and between wealthy and deprived regions and localities. Moreover, it will waste vast amounts of money and increase the pressure and surveillance on those who already feel their lives are pressurised, monitored and controlled. This is not just top-down, explicit control. It is, as Foucault (1979) so powerfully demonstrated, the insinuation of the disciplines of power: naming, framing and blaming the problems and the people and bringing the already limited freedoms of their everyday lives under closer and closer scrutiny and negative comment.

From time to time, we catch glimpses of other ways of addressing health in society: a greater emphasis on primary care; greater secondary care expertise working alongside primary care; unblocking the pathways from secondary care into social care; putting healthy living centres into disadvantaged communities to work with general practitioners and with local communities; supporting community food cooperatives; giving people a greater sense of ownership and control of their services; putting work into workless areas; making the work, tax and benefit systems more flexible; not just talking about partnership, community engagement and sustainability, but doing it.

The weight of the pressures to prevent the formulation and implementation of what seem demonstrably rational policies are considerable. Hospitals as institutions have ways of binding in resources that make well-laid plans for primary care-based systems very difficult to put into practice. Health professionals are often too closely linked to the dominant model of medicine and too detached from economic and regeneration policies to link the health improvement agenda clearly to wider policy agendas. There remain assumptions about knowledge and expertise that are internally contradictory. On the one hand, it is clear that health promotion is not 'rocket science', as the public health minister Caroline Flint remarked about the relationship between diet and obesity, so everyone can do it if they would only try harder. On the other hand, people living in deprived areas are characterised as so unintelligent, ill informed or feckless that they cannot get the message – whatever that message may be. Simple messages: Eat properly! Drink less! Give up smoking! Lose weight! Use a condom!

Developing sustainable health action

New forms of health action are difficult to set up and sustain. In spite of academic and lay knowledge that indicates the wide and complex determinants of people's health problems, there is still a default retreat to medicine, and more medicine, which seems so much easier to cost and measure: numbers of doctors and nurses, available beds, drugs bills and waiting times. It is so much more difficult to conceptualise, let alone examine empirically, social capital, social relationships, local resources, autonomy and control, and how people feel about themselves, the people they live with and the places they inhabit. Although our own everyday experiences suggest that friendship and acquaintance, a sense of pride in place and one's place in a community, and a sense of one's capacity to influence are all crucial to our wellbeing, the pathways to health (especially if seen as the absence of disease) are more difficult to pinpoint and plot. These are very 'holistic' phenomena that do not slot comfortably into the different categories of thought of different disciplines – disciplines that, to the man or woman in the street, on the bus or in the football crowd, may be about very similar kinds of things. The current emphasis on experimental testing of new programmes or policies to produce reliable evidence means that 'uncontrolled' studies that are participative, developmental but demonstrably rational continue to give rise to suspicion both among intellectual positivists and cash-conscious civil servants. The resurgent, positive influence of Donald T. Campbell, whose life's work emphasised the need to develop a policy or reform by 'checking it out' in experimental or quasi-experimental research (1969, 1973), involves a tightly controlled methodology and epistemology that may in fact be of 'limited significance as a general definition of rationality' (Dehue, 2001, p 297).

The projects funded under the SHARP programme have tried in different ways to explore alternatives to what used to be called the 'dominant ideology' of possessive individualism, with its emphases on technology, expertise and capital investment, and its inevitable demands for quick-fix changes in behaviour and improvements in health. They have all emphasised what is sometimes called 'empowerment' (Wallerstein, 2006). They have attempted to 'do' partnership, community engagement and sustainability, and, equally importantly, to examine what works, how it works and what matters to the people concerned. To consider what works without considering what matters and to whom is a recipe for continued failure, not least against the requirements of 'full engagement' articulated most powerfully to policy makers by Derek Wanless (2004). The SHARP projects have attempted only to look at what works if it matters – if it matters to members of the communities with which the projects have engaged.

Demonstrable rationality has to look at questions of value as well as questions of evidence (Rein, 1986). The contexts in which the projects were operating were complex, dynamic and variable. They were communities where there were cases of genuine and absolute material want in which the health and lives of people experiencing such deprivation would be severely damaged by it. But Chapter Eight's graphic account of processes of social exclusion makes clear that they were also situations in which relative and contingent factors served continually to create uncertainty, anxiety and stress, while simultaneously undermining the possibility of people having a say in processes of governance that might help to reduce uncertainty and establish a sense of control. The evidence that arises from action research in such settings is infused with values. The stories people tell about the difference made by their involvement in SHARP, the activities of SHARP and the outcomes of SHARP, felt at individual, family and community levels, do form evidence (Rein, 1986); the case for community-based action is made all the more rational and powerful by its affective and moral base.

As indicated in Chapter Three, the origins of this approach to developing a programme of sustainable health based on action research are not entirely clear. It is certainly the case that from the beginning the Welsh Assembly Government was intent on developing its own approach to health, one that it perceived to be more community-based and public health-orientated than the approach in England. Nonetheless, what SHARP was modelled on is not clear, and there had already been the SARP (Social Action Research Project) and the SAPHC (Strategic Action Programme for Health Promoting Communities) programmes in key sites in England that had attempted similar projects of connecting universities, health agencies and local communities, with mixed results (Pickin et al, 2002). As the chapters in this volume have indicated, SHARP was a bold, complex and multidimensional programme, seeking innovation and learning for policy, with minimal controls over anything beyond the financial viability of the projects. There was support, particularly to help draw out the learning from the projects, but very little attempt directly to influence the intellectual or social trajectories of the projects. There were some attempts to quality assure the projects through the introduction of external evaluators. However, the findings from the external evaluators were used as a way of filling out and broadening the conclusions from the individual projects, rather than acting in any way to direct and control the work that the individual projects were doing. They were allowed to develop criteria of the demonstrably rational among themselves, and the funders and evaluators were understanding of and sympathetic to the complex ways in which evidence and evaluation took place. The main concern for the Welsh Assembly seemed to be not so much whether the projects 'proved' anything in the normally accepted sense of the term, but whether or not the (evidence-based) initiatives they developed were feasible, what the processes of implementation were, what range of impacts could be discerned and whether or in what sense these would be sustainable. The complex issue of sustainability has been discussed elsewhere (Cropper et al, 2007).

Practical utopianism

There are some who will consider all this to be the utopianism of a new government not yet fully connected to the responsibilities of power. But SHARP raises some serious and important questions about the basis of genuine political rationality, and by what metrics success or failure can be measured. In the conclusion to their classic account, Marris and Rein argue:

> Community action set out to change the way problems were perceived, by opening new channels of communication. In this it largely failed, in the short run, because it had no power to alter the priorities of attention. But from its frustrations arose a movement to protest the right of the poor and all politically disadvantaged minorities to be heard, which over the decade has profoundly influenced our conceptions of democracy. (Marris and Rein, 1974, p 364)

What the contributions to this book have shown is that it is possible to establish a rallying point, or catalyst, for work towards a more social or communitarian model of health improvement. The SHARP projects did confirm that it is possible to engage or re-engage with communities that have been defined by public service organisations as problematic, despite, or because of, their need. It is possible to create linkages, to release energies and to create facilities, services, initiatives and action that are valued by communities that had little of any of these things. It is possible to turn resources and attention towards communities for the purposes of health improvement. But such a reorientation is fragile, and requires continued investment, change in organisational cultures, and vigilance with regard to the way in which power is distributed between state and citizens and between professionals and lay people. If the 'priorities of attention' in government and the professions are not changed, it is very difficult for these relatively inexpensive, community-based projects to seem anything other than utopian. However, the frustration and anger that comes from utopia denied is an important component in widening public participation (Elliott and Williams, 2003).

The SHARP programme reflects a considerable commitment in the Welsh Assembly Government to finding ways of building health from the bottom up. And when the opportunity was afforded, the projects showed that, at different speeds and in varying ways, local people and front-line professionals were able and willing to act. There were disadvantages in having the projects linked to institutions of higher education – they sometimes seemed remote, and to be operating with a conventional set of academic standards of project management and targets, driven by the needs of individual academics and the higher educational institution. However, the link to universities was also a source of power. It made it more difficult for the projects to become captured or controlled by either agency or community interests within the localities in which they were operating. While the role of the universities might not always have been entirely clear to those working in the front line in disadvantaged communities, it was certainly the case that universities had an independence from the sometimes intense, local politics that surround any project of this kind. The way in which the projects were funded and set up allowed them to develop a hybrid form that was neither pure 'research' nor pure 'community development', something that very much fits the model of community-based action research. In its various forms, this participative, reflective process allowed the projects to develop activities that were relevant to and, to some extent, driven by local people, but within a framework in which research and evaluation were built into the whole idea of what was to be done.

Modern health and social policies are developed in an environment that is shaped by political, moral and scientific, or at least evidential, claims. The development of increasing concern with the evidence base for policy is to be welcomed, as long as the scientists, policy makers and citizens involved recognise that the process of making policy more evidence-based does not eliminate political interests and moral values. The collection and utilisation of scientific evidence is, by definition, something that is driven by those with the scientific expertise to be able to undertake research and evaluation. However, these developments do not make the construction and implementation of policy any less a moral enterprise than it always has been; judgements of worth, desert or need still have to be made, and the analysis of data does not do this for us:

> It is less threatening to evade the moral issue by treating questions of social action as practical problems with rational solutions, to which reasonable people will agree, once the evidence has been laid out for them. But this, of course, takes for granted the moral assumptions which underlie the way the problem has been set, and the uncertainty of those assumptions is the heart of the difficulty. (Marris, 1996, p 157)

The uncertainty is part of the difficulty of trying to be modern and decisive in policy formation and implementation in a post-modern culture and society, one in which basic assumptions most certainly cannot be assumed to be shared. Many of the projects in the SHARP programme reveal the plurality of views and perspectives that some characterise as 'post-modern' and the way in which this plurality creates opportunities for much richer approaches to problem definition and problem solving.

In the Preface to this book, we noted that there was a commitment to the widest possible dissemination of findings from SHARP and a willingness among the Welsh Assembly Government sponsors of the project to wait for the appropriate moment for findings to be formally reported. Throughout, the projects have sought to influence local policy and practice and, where evaluation has been systematic, have reported through academic and professional literatures. Policy learning has occurred through informal presentations and word-of-mouth conversations within emerging policy communities, with access laterally through other programmes, such as the Health Inequalities Fund, Communities First and the voluntary sector, as well as vertically through the Welsh Assembly Government's Health Promotion Division to the policy lead, the Chief Medical Officer. A year of tapered funding gave the projects time to seek transfer of the resources and activities they saw as being most beneficial; and in many cases, projects, or particular elements of projects, continue, through further short-term monies or through assimilation into mainstream practices. There were also regular meetings of the seven projects and an overarching evaluation project, undertaken by academics at Keele University, to draw out findings from the programme as a whole. Reports of these meetings and of the overarching evaluation carry the detail of SHARP's trials and tribulations.

The policy context in Wales changed during the course of SHARP: in particular, public health, given the strongest mandate through the Wanless Report (Wanless, 2004), was caught by 'politically unfortunate news' about hospital services, at least when access to services was compared with the progress made in England on waiting lists and times. Changes at both ministerial and Chief Medical Officer levels meant that the interest in and commitment to SHARP became less personal. Nevertheless, the wider sets of conclusions have been received in presentations within the Welsh Assembly to ministers, policy makers and programme managers working on the implementation of community policy (for example, Communities First). The impact is not yet clear. An issue has been to find an appropriate 'level of resolution' for the findings: good specific ideas that go with the grain of policy and add to the list of 'good practice ideas' may be enthusiastically received; broader findings that cross government policy lines may be less easily given and assimilated. For example, there is question about where the policy lead on health inequalities, viewed as the cross-cutting wider determinants of health, would best be located – in health and social care or, for example, in social justice and regeneration, under which banner the Welsh community development and regeneration programme Communities First is located. In Chapter Eight, Robert Moore notes the way in which policies and the 'rules' they mandate can fail to square. The contrast between involvement in SHARP and the experience of Communities First was stark for some active members of communities and there is a question about *how* community-led partnerships are expected or required to demonstrate good governance and performance.

Locally, there has been both enthusiasm and resistance to the dissemination of lessons from SHARP in equal measure. SHARP, with projects established mostly as 'joint ventures' outside the mainstream service agencies, had choices about where to locate its efforts to support and influence local agencies. But where the clearest choice was not fully receptive, the project may also end up outside the system 'shouting in', or, at best, seeking to work around the official gatekeepers and through more sympathetic informal routes. Evidence may count less than the 'practical technologies' developed and tested by SHARP and left behind as 'going concerns' and 'assets': the package of measures needed to maintain swimming sessions for women, the idea of a community researcher or programme of community-resourced research, peer counselling in schools, the 'community house' as a focus for community activities and deliberations, and a youth forum or council, as examples. Participants' personal testaments revealed how SHARP had helped individuals, families and communities to change the way they viewed themselves and also demonstrated a return of 'hope' (Baum, 1997). But we also saw, in equal measure, the realpolitik of community and democratic leadership. SHARP was seen as 'parachuted' in and the local agencies then left to find ways of maintaining the effort, or to decide not to provide support. The specific resources and activities supported by SHARP can, at least, be maintained where they are seen as providing value. Whether the ethos and practices of co-inquiry that brought them into being can be maintained is another matter.

We have referred to the concept of 'demonstrable rationality' in policy as one that is in many ways preferable to the notion of policy being evidence-based. It suggests something that involves a synthesis of ideas, information and perspectives (as Carlisle and colleagues in Chapter Seven note, Weiss (1991) talks of ideas, facts and arguments) whose use can be demonstrated, rather than implying that there is a study or body of evidence that can be referred to as true in some way that suggests the science can make decisions for us. Many of the approaches to systematic reviews of literature in the area of health and social interventions now recognise that it is not enough to review studies within some kind of hierarchy of evidence when there is no agreement on what the 'priorities of attention' are in the issues being examined. Many concepts, decisions and strategies for implementation, including health inequalities, social inclusion and social capital, are *essentially* contested. In the modern world, there are many people who consider themselves to be perfectly reasonable and rational, contesting things strenuously with other people, who also believe themselves to be reasonable and rational, and who contest equally strenuously.

For all this, however, policy makers will still need evidence that can in some sense be presented as reliable, sound and robust. Some may argue that the whole point and basis of the movement to make medicine, healthcare and health policy more evidence-based is that it will reduce the number and intensity of areas of decision making that are essentially contested. More and better sources of evidence can act as tools for thinking and decision making, but evidence will still provoke different interpretations based on meaning structures:

> The conflict between incompatible meanings cannot be resolved simply by producing evidence, not because evidence is irrelevant, but because its relevance can only be determined by the meanings themselves. (Marris, 1996, p 31)

In a local and inevitably circumscribed way, SHARP allowed for more fluid and contextualised forms of demonstrable rationality to emerge from a social process of partnership and participation. At the most basic level, it showed how the process of collecting and analysing evidence in communities of the kind that the projects worked in could be successfully and creatively done by members of the community themselves. In some cases, these were ordinary, unpaid, volunteer community members. In others, local people were recruited as paid 'community researchers'. None was a 'usual suspect' or established community leader. Many stuck with the project from start to finish and continue to work in a community-based role. In each case, they worked with others, or took the findings to others, from health and local government agencies and from universities, which brought different meanings to the process. As many of the reports on the projects make clear, the incompatibility of meanings was not something comfortable and soft, but often discomforting, hard and sharp. Nor was the creation of alternative routes for direct community representation and advocacy always readily accepted. In other words, this was no easy, consensus-based approach to the generation and implementation of knowledge, within an action research cycle. It was about the generation of new evidence, but within a process of democratic enrichment that allowed different meaning structures to be used and themselves tested.

The action research projects provided a framework in which the negotiation of the meanings of the evidence gathered could be undertaken in a manner that allowed sustained inquiry. Commonly, consultation with communities would be a short-run measure, repeated as agencies saw fit or were required to demonstrate, the findings owned by the agencies and with no community right to reply. The SHARP projects vested the evidence in their communities and supported processes of evidence gathering and analysis, sense making and use, including advocacy and voice: as Chapter Seven indicates, evidence *for* change could be powerful and not just in contexts that are wholly sympathetic to the privilege given to community-expressed needs and preferences.

Evidence, in itself, does not produce innovation; and many of the actions undertaken through or as a consequence of SHARP projects were not, in themselves, innovative. The range of action is perhaps unusual for a health programme – film club, online poetry and literature, driving lessons for young men, training in car mechanics for young women, women-only swimming classes, a walking club, a food cooperative, an event celebrating diverse food cultures, a youth council for a town, basketball, exercise classes in a community hall. More unusual, however, is that these were all developed by and with members of communities for their communities. And in some cases, the process of development continued. Women who had negotiated the right to single-gender swimming classes asked to be trained as lifeguards and subsequently became employed as such.

The projects have also produced knowledge and learning – evidence *about* action and the significance of changes that have been experienced in the communities where action has been rooted. They have done this in three main ways. First, they have shown how to translate the phrase 'action to address health inequalities' into meaningful practical action that can help justify and lever investment. This has led to new facilities (spaces to meet, CCTV), community resources and activities (film club, educational programme, exercise class, community forum), and to changes in local social relationships, a release of community capacity, and individual development and community strengthening. Second, in relation to partnership and institutional change, the projects have demonstrated how, even with 'full engagement' by local communities, resistance among professionals and institutions, sometimes because of the other pressures they face, make changes in organisational culture and practice a real impediment to sustainable transformation (Pickin et al, 2002). Finally, they have shown how action research can act as a lever to bind a range of interests into a process of co-inquiry, matched by commitments within a programme of action, that offers the promise of taking us beyond limited conceptions of evidence and experiment to meaningful and demonstrable rationality.

References

Adler, P. and Kwon, S.-W. (2002) 'Social capital: prospects for a new concept', *Academy of Management Review*, vol 27, pp 17-40.

Bardach, E. (1998) *Getting Agencies to Work Together: The Practice and Theory of Managerial Craftsmanship*, Washington, DC: Brookings Institution Press.

Baum, H. (1997) *The Organization of Hope*, Albany, NY: University of New York Press.

Bloor, M. (2000) 'The South Wales Miners Federation, miners' lung and the instrumental use of expertise, 1900-1950', *Social Studies of Science*, vol 30, pp 124-40.

Campbell, D.T. (1969) 'Reforms as experiments', *American Psychologist*, vol 24, p 409-29.

Campbell, D.T. (1974) 'The social scientist as methodological servant of the experimenting society', *Policy Studies Journal*, vol 2, pp 72-5.

Cornwall, R. (2007) 'Learning, soft skills and community regeneration: a case study analysis', Unpublished PhD thesis, School of Social Sciences, Cardiff University.

Cropper, S. (2002) 'What contributions might ideas of social capital make to policy implementation for reducing health inequalities?', Paper to Health Development Agency Seminar Series, Tackling Health Inequalities: Turning Policy into Practice. Seminar 3: Organisational Change and Systems Management, London: Royal Aeronautical Society, 17 September (www.nice.org.uk/page.aspx?o=508190).

Cropper, S., Carlisle, S., Beech, R. and Little, R. (2007) *The Sustainability and Transferability of SHARP: Report to Welsh Assembly Government*, Keele: Keele University.

Dehue, T. (2001) 'Establishing the experimenting society: the historical origin of social experimentation according to the randomized controlled design', *American Journal of Psychology*, vol 114, pp 283-302.

Dennett, J., James, E., Room, G. and Watson, P. (1982) *Europe Against Poverty: The European Poverty Programme 1975-1980*, London: Bedford Square Press.

Elliott, E. and Williams, G. (2003) 'Developing a civic intelligence: local involvement in health impact assessment', *Environmental Impact Assessment Review*, vol 24, pp 231-43.

Exworthy, M. and Powell, M. (2000, unpublished) 'Understanding health variations and policy variations', ESRC End of Award Report, L128231039.

Exworthy, M., Berney, L. and Powell, M. (2002) 'How great expectations in Westminster may be dashed locally – the local implementation of national policy on health inequalities', *Policy and Politics*, vol 30, pp 79-96.

Foucault, M. (1979) *The Birth of the Clinic*, Harmondsworth: Penguin.

Francis, H. and Smith, D. (1998) *The Fed: A History of the South Wales Miners in the Twentieth Century* (centenary edn), Cardiff: University of Wales Press.

Goodwin, M. and Armstrong-Esther, D. (2004) 'Children, social capital and health: Increasing the well-being of young people in rural Wales', *Children's Geographies*, vol 2, no 1, pp 49-63.

Gorman, R.A. (1995) *Michael Harrington: Speaking American*, London: Routledge.

Harrington, M. (1971) *The Other America: Poverty in the United States*, Harmondsworth: Penguin.

Huxham, C. and Vangen, S. (2005) *Managing to Collaborate: The Theory and Practice of Collaborative Advantage*, Abingdon: Routledge.

Jasanoff, S. (2007) *Designs on Nature: Science and Democracy in Europe and the United States*, Princeton, NJ: Princeton University Press.

Jones, R.M. (1982) *The North Wales Quarrymen, 1874-1922*, Cardiff: University of Wales Press.

Levitas, R. (1998) *The Inclusive Society? Social Exclusion and New Labour*, Basingstoke: Palgrave.

Lowndes, V. and Wilson, D. (2001) 'Social capital and local governance: exploring the institutional design variable', *Political Studies*, vol 49, pp 629-47.

Marris, P. (1996) *The Politics of Uncertainty: Attachment in Public and Private Life*, London: Routledge.

Marris, P. and Rein, M. (1974) *Dilemmas of Social Reform* (2nd edn), Harmondsworth: Penguin.

Nahapiet, J. and Ghoshal, S. (1998) 'Social capital, intellectual capital and the organisational advantage', *Academy of Management Review*, vol 23, no 2, pp 242-66.

Nutley, S., Walter, I. and Davies, H.W.O (2007) *Using Evidence: How Research can Inform Public Services*, Bristol: The Policy Press.

Pickin, C., Popay, J., Staley, K., Bruce, N., Jones, C. and Gowman, N. (2002) 'Developing a model to enhance the capacity of statutory organisations to engage with lay communities', *Journal of Health Services Research & Policy*, vol 7, pp 34-42.

Pope, R. (1998) *Building Jerusalem: Nonconformity, Labour and the Social Question in Wales, 1906-1939*, Cardiff: University of Wales Press

Rein, M. (1986) *Social Science and Public Policy*, Harmondsworth: Penguin.

Smith, D. (1993) *Aneurin Bevan and the World of South Wales*, Cardiff: University of Wales Press.

Sullivan, H. and Skelcher, C.(2002) *Working across Boundaries: Collaboration in Public Services*, Basingstoke: Palgrave Macmillan.

Wallerstein, N. (2006) *What is the evidence on effectiveness of empowerment to improve health?* Copenhagen: WHO Regional Office for Europe (Health Evidence Network report, accessed 01 February 2006).

Wanless, D (2004) *Securing Good Health for the Whole Population: Final Report* (the Wanless Report), London: HM Treasury.

Weiss, C.H. (1991) 'Policy research: data, ideas or arguments', in P. Wagner, C.H. Weiss, B. Wittrock and H. Wolman (eds) *Social Science and Modern States*, Cambridge: Cambridge University Press.

Welsh Office (1998) *Better Health – Better Wales*, Cm 3922, Cardiff: The Stationery Office.

Woolcock, M. (2001) 'The place of social capital in understanding social and economic outcomes', *Canadian Journal of Policy Research*, vol 2, no 1, pp 11-17.

Index

SHARP DVD
A Way of Working Together to Improve Our Lives

Lessons from the Sustainable Health Action Research Programme (SHARP) in Wales

The Sustainable Health Action Research Programme (SHARP) was an action research initiative focusing on community health development, funded by the Welsh Assembly Government between 2000 and 2006. Adopting an action research approach, the initiative encouraged partnerships consisting of public, private, voluntary and academic sectors to work with local communities in tackling locally identified issues impacting on people's health and wellbeing.

The DVD was produced to further disseminate the learning from SHARP. It captures what evolved from this six-year programme through the voices of members of seven projects across Wales. The DVD also provides practical examples on how to undertake action research, drawing on the experiences of SHARP. The key messages from the DVD include:

- The importance of health determinants and the broad context of policies addressing health and wellbeing e.g. education, access to leisure/sport activities, equality, young people and children, housing, social inclusion and community regeneration.
- The need to develop local solutions to local problems through active community involvement.
- The potential of the community-based action research approach.
- The importance of partnership working and the challenges that this can pose.
- Community engagement that goes beyond consultation.
- The importance of legacy and sustainability i.e. looking beyond the funding period from the earliest stages of a programme.

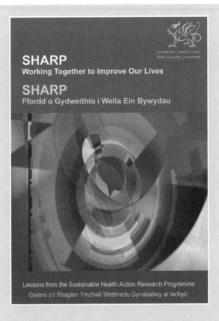

The film is produced in English and Welsh, with optional subtitles. From the Main Menu screen viewers can choose nine sections, as follows:

- Main film 'What we learnt from SHARP' (approximately 21 minutes long).
- Snapshot of project (7 sections, each section approximately 4 to 8 minutes long).

If you'd like to obtain copies of the DVD please email sharp@wales.gsi.gov.uk, providing your name, postal address, telephone number and number of copies you wish to receive. Further information on SHARP can be found at SHARP website: www.wales.gov.uk/cmoresearch (English) or www.cymru.gov.uk/ymchwilcmo (Welsh).

Contact: Kaori Onoda
Research and Evaluation
Department for Public Health and Health Professions
Welsh Assembly Government
Cathays Park
Cardiff CF10 3NQ
UK